MOSBY'S COMPREHENSIVE PHYSICAL THERAPIST ASSISTANT BOARD REVIEW

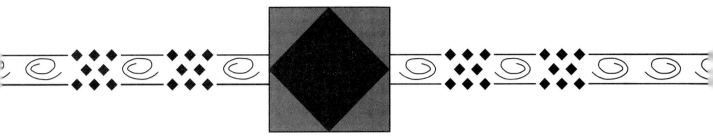

MOSBY'S COMPREHENSIVE PHYSICAL THERAPIST ASSISTANT BOARD REVIEW

Shirley J. Brister, M.A., R.P.T.

Administrator,
HEALTHSOUTH Sports Medicine and Rehabilitation Center;
Adjunct Faculty Member,
Physical Therapist Assistant Program,
Tulsa Junior College,
Tulsa, Oklahoma

with 222 illustrations

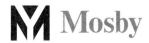 Mosby

St. Louis Baltimore Boston Carlsbad Chicago Naples New York Philadelphia Portland
London Madrid Mexico City Singapore Sydney Tokyo Toronto Wiesbaden

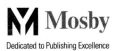

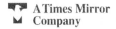

Executive Editor: Martha Sasser
Developmental Editor: Kellie F. White
Project Manager: Peggy Fagen
Manufacturing Supervisor: Karen Lewis
Editing and Production: Top Graphics
Designer: Sheilah Barrett

Printed in the United States of America
Composition by Top Graphics
Printing/binding by William C. Brown

Mosby–Year Book, Inc.
11830 Westline Industrial Drive
St. Louis, Missouri 63146

Library of Congress Cataloging-in-Publication Data

Brister, Shirley J.
    Mosby's comprehensive physical therapist assistant board review /
Shirley J. Brister.
        p.   cm.
    Includes bibliographical references and index.
    ISBN 0-8151-1010-3
    1. Physical therapy—Outlines, syllabi, etc.   2. Physical therapy—
Examinations, questions, etc.   3. Physical therapy assistants.
I. Title.
    [DNLM: 1. Physical Therapy—outlines.   2. Physical Therapy—
examination questions.   3. Allied Health Personnel.   WB 18.2 B861m
1995]
RM701.6.B75   1995
615.8′2′076—dc20
DNLM/DLC
for Library of Congress   95-31273
                                                             CIP

95 96 97 98 99 / 9 8 7 6 5 4 3 2 1

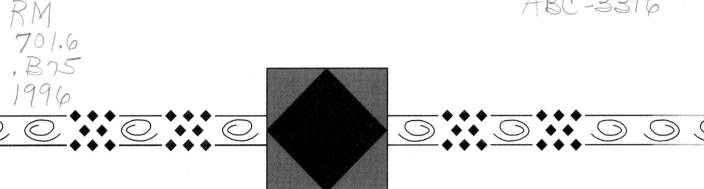

To my aunt, Florence Pevehouse, who encouraged
me in setting and achieving both professional and
personal goals in my life

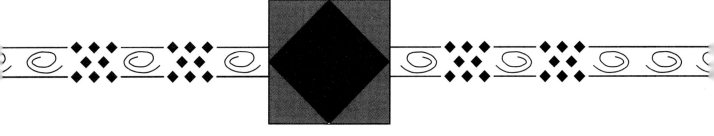

Preface

In the spring of 1994, the second-year physical therapist assistant students at Tulsa Junior College asked if I would help them review for their board examination. After several weeks of searching for a textbook, I discovered that one did not exist in the format that we desired. Thus began the process of filling that void.

The information presented in *Mosby's Comprehensive Physical Therapist Assistant Board Review* was written to prepare physical therapist assistants for the ultimate educational achievement—passing their board examination. This book may also be used as a refresher guide by practicing physical therapist assistants.

The curricula of over 30 physical therapist assistant programs across the country were researched during the formation of this textbook. Each chapter covers one area of study, beginning with an overview of the subject matter and closing with a series of review questions to test knowledge and comprehension. An answer key and blank answer sheets follow each review section. In addition, for easy reference, a comprehensive glossary is included at the back of the book. Through the course of this book, you will review:

- Medical terminology
- Medicolegal issues
- Anatomy, physiology, and kinesiology
- Neuroanatomy and neurology
- Common diagnoses in physical therapy, including orthopedic disorders, neurological disorders, pulmonary disorders, and burns
- Common psychological disorders
- Pediatric growth and development and the neurological assessment of children
- Therapeutic modalities used in physical therapy
- Therapeutic exercise

You will find that the order of the topics presented is based on standard physical therapist assistant curriculum. Unlike many board reviews, your study with this book is supplemented by numerous illustrations. You will find these visual aids most helpful in your review of anatomy, physiology, and kinesiology.

Included with this text are two practice examinations, which should be very similar to the board examination you are preparing to take. These practice examinations will help you to move from studying specific topics to taking a comprehensive look at and review of your past 2 years of education.

I wish you the best of luck in preparing for and passing your physical therapist assistant board examination.

Shirley J. Brister, M.A., R.P.T.

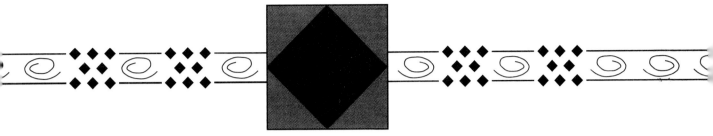

Acknowledgments

First and foremost, I would like to express my appreciation to my aunt, Florence Pevehouse, for her endless support and prayers over the years. She provided me a hideout several times in the past year to write and compile my thoughts. Also I want to thank Jo Harvey, Linda Colvard, and Karen Waite for their encouragement, love, and patience during the past year as I have written this book.

A very special thank you goes to the greatest editing staff in the world: Martha Sasser, Kellie White, and Amy Dubin. As a first-time author, I will always appreciate the encouragement and guidance they so patiently gave me.

I want to extend my thanks to the doctors at Central States Orthopaedics for whom I worked for 12 glorious years. In addition, I want to thank Patricia Thomas for her professional and personal encouragement and challenge to reach higher and strive for the best.

Special recognition and thanks go to the Tulsa Junior College Physical Therapist Assistant Class of 1994 who gave me the opportunity to experiment with a very rough format of this book during a review course for their board examination.

Special thanks also go to the faculty members of the Physical Therapist Assistant Program at Tulsa Junior College. As an adjunct faculty member to the program, I appreciate Suzanne Reese, Kathy Johnson, and Carla Hinkle for their encouragement, support, and suggestions.

Thanks also to Brad Harvey, graphic artist, for his assistance with the illustrations.

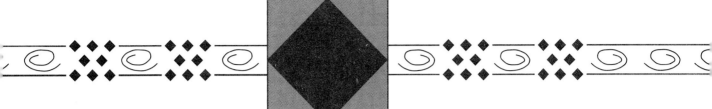

Contents

MOSBY'S COMPREHENSIVE PHYSICAL THERAPIST ASSISTANT BOARD REVIEW

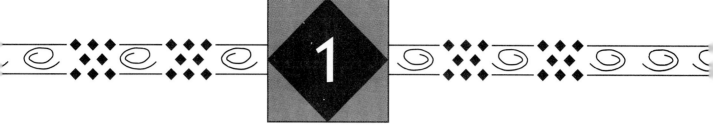

Medical Terminology

Medical terminology is the study of terminology used in all areas of medical science and paramedical specialties. A basic understanding of medical words can be gained by recognizing their Latin and Greek parts. Reviewing the most common root words, suffixes, prefixes, and medical abbreviations is the first step in your review process.

GLOSSARY OF WORD PARTS

Word Part	Meaning	Example
a-	without	apnea
ab-	deviating from	abnormal
abdomin/o-	abdomen	abdominocentesis
acid	sour	acidosis
acr/o-	extremity	acromegaly
acromi/o-	acromion	acromiohumeral
acu-	needle	acupressure
ad-	toward	adduction
aden/o-	gland	adenectomy
adip-	fat	adipose
aer/o-	air	aerotherapy
alges/i-	oversensitivity to pain	analgesia
-algia	pain	cardialgia
amb/i-	both sides	ambidextrous
an-	without	anesthesia
angi/o-	vessel	angiofibroma
anis/o-	unequal	anisocytosis
ankyl/o-	stiff	anklyosis
ante-	before	antepyretic
anti-	against	antiseptic
antr-	cavern, sinus	antrum
appendic/o-	appendix	appendicitis
arteri/o-	artery	arteriosclerosis
arthr/o-	joint	arthritis
audi/o-	hear, hearing	audiometer
aut/o-	self	autophobia
bi-	two, double	biceps
bi/o-	life	biology
bil/i-	bile	biliuria
blast/o-	cell	myoblast

Word Part	Meaning	Example
brachi/o-	upper arm	brachialgia
brady-	slow	bradycardia
bronch/o-	bronchi	bronchitis
burs/o-	bursa	bursitis
calcane/o-	heel	calcanodynia
carcin/o-	cancer	carcinoma
cardi/o-	heart	megalocardia
carp/o-	wrist	carpectomy
caud/o-	toward the tail	caudad
-cele	herniation	encephalocele
cephal/o-	toward the head	cephalalgia
cerebr-	cerebrum	craniocerebral
chir/o-	hand	chirospasm
chondr/o-	cartilage	chondrectomy
circum-	around	circumduction
cleid/o-	clavicle	sternocleidomastoid
con-	with	congenital
condyl/o-	rounded process	epicondyle
contra-	against	contraindication
cortic/o-	cortex	cortical
cost/o-	rib	costovertebral
cox-	hip joint	coxa vara
crani/o-	skull	craniectomy
cry/o-	cold	cryotherapy
cyan/o	blue	cyanosis
dactyl-	digit	macrodactylia
derm/o-	skin	dermatitis
dis-	apart, separation	dislocate
dynam-	power, strength	dynamometer
-dynia	pain	cephalodynia
dys-	difficult	dyspnea
ect/o-	outer	ectoderm
-ectomy	removal	gastrectomy
edema	swelling	pseudoedema
emesis	vomiting	hyperemesis
-emia	blood	erythremia
encephal/o-	brain	encephalitis
epi-	over, upon	epidural
erythr/o-	red	erythropsia
extra-	outside	extraarticular
faci-	face	facial
fasci-	band, fascia	myofascial
femor/o-	femur	pubofemoral
fibr/o-	fiber	neurofibroma
gangli/o-	nerve cell	ganglion
gastr/o-	stomach	gastrointestinal
genu-	knee	genu varum
gluteo-	buttock	gluteus maximus
goni/o-	angle	goniometer
graph/o-	record	electrocardiograph
hem/o-	blood	hemarthrosis
hemi-	half	hemiplegia
hist-	tissue	histology
hydr/o-	water	hydrotherapy

Word Part	Meaning	Example
hyper-	above, more than	hypertrophy
hypo-	under, less than	hypotrophy
in-	in, not	incompetence
infra-	below, under	infrapatellar
intra-	within	intraabdominal
ischi/o-	ischium	ischiopubic
-itis	inflammation	arthritis
kine-	movement, motion	kinesiology
later/o-	side	anterolateral
lumb/o-	loin	lumbosacral
lys/o-	destruction of	neurolysis
macr/o-	large, enlarge	macrocyte
mal-	bad, abnormal	malformation
malac/o-	softening	chondromalacia
medi-	middle	mediastinum
megal-	large	megalocardia
mening/o-	membrane	meningitis
mes/o-	middle	mesoderm
my/o-	muscle	myocarditis
myel/o-	spinal cord	myelocele
neur/o-	nerve cell	neuroblast
-oma	tumor	adenoma
-opia	vision	diplopia
-osis	condition	arteriosclerosis
oste/o-	bone	osteomalacia
par/o-	to bear	multipara
paralysis	loss of movement	acroparalysis
path/o-	disease	adenopathy
-penia	decrease in	leukocytopenia
phalang/o-	finger, toe	phalangectomy
-plasty	repair	cranioplasty
pleur/o-	lung, rib, side	pleuralgia
pneo-	breath	bradypnea
pneum/o-	lung, rib, side	pneumothorax
pod/o-	foot	podalgia
poly-	many	polyuria
post-	after, behind	postoperative
postero-	behind	posterior
pre-	before	prenatal
pro-	before	prognosis
pseud/o-	false	pseudoparalysis
psych/o-	mind	psychoanalysis
ptosis	prolapse	hysteroptosis
pub/o-	pubis	suprapubis
pulmo-	lung	cardiopulmonary
rachi/o-	spine	rachitis
rect/o-	rectum	rectocele
-rrhagia	hemorrhage	pneumonorrhagia
scapul/o-	scapula	scapulothoracic
scler/o-	hardening	arteriosclerosis
scolio-	twisted	scoliosis
semi-	half	semiconscious
spasm/o-	tightening	myospasm
spondyl/o-	spine	spondylitis

Word Part	Meaning	Example
sten/o-	narrow	stenosis
stern/o-	breast bone	sternocleidomastoid
sub-	under	substernal
supra-	above	supraspinatus
tachy-	fast, rapid	tachycardia
therap/o-	treatment	hydrotherapy
therm/o-	heat	thermometer
thorac/o-	chest	thoracotomy
thromb/o-	clot	thrombolysis
-tome	instrument for cutting, piece cut off	dermatome
trache/o-	trachea	tracheotomy
trans-	across	transposition
tri-	three	triceps
uni-	one	unilateral
ultra-	beyond	ultrasound
vas/o-	vessel	vasospasm

MEDICAL ABBREVIATIONS

Abbreviation	Definition
a.c.	before meals
a.j.	ankle jerk
A & P	auscultation and percussion
AP	anteroposterior
b.i.d.	twice a day
B.P.	blood pressure
c	with
C	centigrade
Ca	cancer
cbc	complete blood count
cc	cubic centimeter
C.C.	chief complaint
CCU	cardiac care unit
cm	centimeter
cu	cubic
CVA	cerebrovascular accident
ECG	electrocardiogram
EEG	electroencephalogram
EMG	electromyography
F	Fahrenheit
f.h.s.	fetal heart sounds
f.h.t.	fetal heart tones
G.B.	gallbladder
GI	gastrointestinal
gm	gram
gr	grain
hb	hemoglobin
h.s.	at bedtime
hypo	hypodermically
ICU	intensive care unit
I.M.	intramuscular
I.V.	intravenous
kg	kilogram

Abbreviation	Definition
KUB	kidney, ureter, and bladder
L	liter
LLQ	left lower quadrant
LRQ	lower right quadrant
LUQ	left upper quadrant
mcg	microgram
mg	milligram
mg%	milligram percent
mm	millimeter
ml	milliliter
MRI	magnetic resonance imaging
O_2	oxygen
O.P.D.	out-patient department
O.R.	operating room
oz	ounce
P.	pulse
PA	posteroanterior
P.A.	pernicious anemia
P & A	percussion and auscultation
p.c.	after meals
P.E.	physical examination
P.I.	present illness
p.o.	postoperative or by mouth
p.r.n.	as needed
P.T.	physical therapy
q.	every
q.h.	every hour
q.2h.	every 2 hours
q.i.d.	four times a day
q.m.	every morning
q.n.	every night
R.	respiration
rbc	red blood cells
Rh	blood factor
RLQ	right lower quadrant
RUQ	right upper quadrant
Rx	take
s	without
S.C.	subcutaneously
sed. rate	sedimentation rate
ss	one half
sp. gr.	specific gravity
staph.	staphylococcus
stat.	immediately
strep.	streptococcus
T.	temperature
t.i.d.	three times a day
T.P.R.	temperature, pulse, and respirations
U	unit
ULQ	upper left quadrant
URQ	upper right quadrant
wbc	white blood cells; white blood count

REVIEW QUESTIONS

1. The word root used to form words referring to the extremities is:
   a. ext-
   b. trem-
   c. acr/o-
   d. -ties

2. A prefix meaning "toward" is:
   a. ab-
   b. ex-
   c. ante-
   d. ad-

3. *A-* is a prefix meaning:
   a. With
   b. Without
   c. Before
   d. Toward

4. A word root meaning "with" is:
   a. con-
   b. contra-
   c. cox-
   d. an-

Match the following word roots with the correct meanings:

_____ 5. anti-	a. life	
_____ 6. antr-	b. two	
_____ 7. anis/o-	c. against	
_____ 8. bi-	d. unequal	
_____ 9. bi/o-	e. herniation	
_____ 10. -cele	f. difficult	
_____ 11. dys-	g. sinus	

12. "Acromegaly" means that the extremities are:
    a. Painful
    b. Atrophied
    c. Enlarged
    d. Infected

13. The word root *alges/i-* means:
    a. Number
    b. Numb
    c. Oversensitivity to pain
    d. Against

14. A word part meaning "before" is:
    a. ante-
    b. anti-
    c. be-
    d. angi/o-

15. The word part *ankyl/o-* means:
    a. Ankle
    b. Stiff
    c. Joint
    d. None of the above

16. *Adip-* is a word part meaning:
    a. Fat
    b. Tissue
    c. Air
    d. Face

17. The word part *cry/o-* means:
    a. Tear
    b. Cold
    c. Heat
    d. Over

18. The prefix *caud/o-* means:
    a. Close
    b. Head
    c. Toward the tail
    d. Remove

19. The suffix *-ectomy* means:
    a. Removal
    b. Against
    c. Around
    d. Incision

20. The word root *chondr/o-* means:
    a. Ligament
    b. Tendon
    c. Cartilage
    d. Joint

21. The prefix *dis-* means:
    a. Difficult
    b. Separation
    c. Apart
    d. b and c

22. The word part *circum-* means:
    a. Give up
    b. Below
    c. Around
    d. Beside

23. A word root meaning "over" is:
    a. -emia
    b. epi-
    c. cox-
    d. emesis

24. A word part meaning "cell" is:
    a. -cyst
    b. blast/o-
    c. -emia
    d. None of the above
25. A word part meaning "upper arm" is:
    a. brachi/o-
    b. hum-
    c. cox-
    d. rad-
26. A word part meaning "slow" is:
    a. tachy-
    b. brachi/o-
    c. brady-
    d. hist-
27. A prefix meaning "middle" is:
    a. medi-
    b. endo-
    c. mes/o-
    d. a and c
28. A suffix meaning "inflammation" is:
    a. ischi/o-
    b. -itis
    c. -osis
    d. -opia
29. The word root *genu-* means:
    a. Hip
    b. With
    c. Knee
    d. Lateral
30. A prefix meaning "within" is:
    a. intra-
    b. infra-
    c. pre-
    d. poly-
31. A word part meaning "tumor" is:
    a. fibr/o-
    b. mal-
    c. -oma
    d. a and c
32. A blue discoloration of the skin is:
    a. Acrocyanosis
    b. Acrodermatitis
    c. Cyanoderma
    d. Dermatosis
    e. Leukoderma

33. Low blood pressure is known as:
    a. Hypertension
    b. Cyanosis
    c. Bradycardia
    d. Hypotension
34. A word root meaning "softening" is:
    a. arthr/o-
    b. chondr/o-
    c. dento-
    d. malac/o-
    e. scler/o-
35. A combining form meaning "joint" is:
    a. arthr/o-
    b. chondr/o-
    c. malac/o-
    d. cost/o-
    e. aden/o-
36. As a suffix, *-emia* refers to a condition of:
    a. Blood
    b. Urine
    c. Deficiency
    d. Surplus
    e. Discharge

Match the following abbreviations and definitions:

_____ 37. CVA
_____ 38. C
_____ 39. c
_____ 40. a.c.
_____ 41. AP
_____ 42. b.i.d.
_____ 43. cc
_____ 44. gr
_____ 45. h.s.
_____ 46. gm
_____ 47. L
_____ 48. q.i.d.
_____ 49. Rh
_____ 50. mm
_____ 51. ml
_____ 52. PA
_____ 53. P.A.
_____ 54. P.
_____ 55. q.
_____ 56. s
_____ 57. P & A
_____ 58. p.c.
_____ 59. p.r.n.
_____ 60. q.h.
_____ 61. p.o.
_____ 62. Rx

a. without
b. with
c. centigrade
d. twice a day
e. liter
f. gram
g. at bedtime
h. millimeter
i. milliliter
j. four times a day
k. before meals
l. anteroposterior
m. posteroanterior
n. pernicious anemia
o. percussion and auscultation
p. pulse
q. cubic centimeter
r. grain
s. every
t. cerebrovascular accident
u. blood factor
v. after meals
w. take
x. as needed
y. by mouth
z. every hour

SUGGESTED READINGS

Blauvelt CT, Nelson FRT: *A manual of orthopaedic terminology*, St Louis, 1990, Mosby.
Chabner D: *The language of medicine*, Philadelphia, 1985, WB Saunders.
LaFleur M: *Exploring medical language*, St Louis,1985, Mosby.
Sloane SB: *The medical word book*, Philadelphia, 1973, WB Saunders.
Smith GL, Davis PE: *Medical terminology*, New York, 1993, Wiley.

EXAMINATION ANSWER KEY

1. c	**20.** c	**39.** b	**58.** v
2. d	**21.** d	**40.** k	**59.** x
3. b	**22.** c	**41.** l	**60.** z
4. a	**23.** b	**42.** d	**61.** y
5. c	**24.** b	**43.** q	**62.** w
6. g	**25.** a	**44.** r	
7. d	**26.** c	**45.** g	
8. b	**27.** d	**46.** f	
9. a	**28.** b	**47.** e	
10. e	**29.** c	**48.** j	
11. f	**30.** a	**49.** u	
12. c	**31.** c	**50.** h	
13. c	**32.** c	**51.** i	
14. a	**33.** d	**52.** m	
15. b	**34.** d	**53.** n	
16. a	**35.** a	**54.** p	
17. b	**36.** a	**55.** s	
18. c	**37.** t	**56.** a	
19. a	**38.** c	**57.** o	

EXAMINATION ANSWER SHEET

1. _____	20. _____	39. _____	58. _____
2. _____	21. _____	40. _____	59. _____
3. _____	22. _____	41. _____	60. _____
4. _____	23. _____	42. _____	61. _____
5. _____	24. _____	43. _____	62. _____
6. _____	25. _____	44. _____	
7. _____	26. _____	45. _____	
8. _____	27. _____	46. _____	
9. _____	28. _____	47. _____	
10. _____	29. _____	48. _____	
11. _____	30. _____	49. _____	
12. _____	31. _____	50. _____	
13. _____	32. _____	51. _____	
14. _____	33. _____	52. _____	
15. _____	34. _____	53. _____	
16. _____	35. _____	54. _____	
17. _____	36. _____	55. _____	
18. _____	37. _____	56. _____	
19. _____	38. _____	57. _____	

EXAMINATION ANSWER SHEET

1. _____	20. _____	39. _____	58. _____
2. _____	21. _____	40. _____	59. _____
3. _____	22. _____	41. _____	60. _____
4. _____	23. _____	42. _____	61. _____
5. _____	24. _____	43. _____	62. _____
6. _____	25. _____	44. _____	
7. _____	26. _____	45. _____	
8. _____	27. _____	46. _____	
9. _____	28. _____	47. _____	
10. _____	29. _____	48. _____	
11. _____	30. _____	49. _____	
12. _____	31. _____	50. _____	
13. _____	32. _____	51. _____	
14. _____	33. _____	52. _____	
15. _____	34. _____	53. _____	
16. _____	35. _____	54. _____	
17. _____	36. _____	55. _____	
18. _____	37. _____	56. _____	
19. _____	38. _____	57. _____	

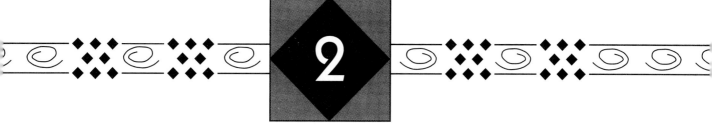

Introduction to Physical Therapy

DOCUMENTATION

In the rehabilitation of patients it is important to record information in a manner that enables other health care professionals and third-party payers (insurance companies) to interpret it easily. As the dollars for health care become less available, payers in the health care system are focusing more on the concept of outcomes management. Many insurance companies are convinced that the relationship between medical treatment intervention and functional outcome must be a priority in their reimbursement decisions.

The most efficient method to demonstrate such outcomes or improvement is the health care provider's documentation in the patient's medical record.[1] Therefore proper documentation in the medical record is vital to demonstrate that the services rendered were medically necessary, had a reasonable potential to result in significant improvement, and were provided as billed.[2]

One of the more common recording methods developed by Lawrence L. Weed is the problem-oriented medical record (POMR), which uses "SOAP" notes.[2] This method of documentation can be used for all patients evaluated and treated in the physical therapy clinic. The most important function of SOAP notes is the improvement of patient care.

SOAP is an acronym in which the letters stand for:

S = subjective
O = objective
A = assessment
P = plan

Subjective: This portion contains the patient's past medical history and present complaint or symptoms. It refers to the information the patient communicates directly to the therapist or assistant.

Objective: This portion contains the data or signs the therapist or assistant observes. It also is a summary of all the clinical tests and treatments that the therapist and assistant perform (e.g., muscle testing, range of motion, functional testing, and manual procedures). This part of the evaluation has been called the looking phase.

Assessment: In this portion the therapist or assistant expresses a professional opinion. A list of problems found in the subjective and objective portions and a working diagnosis should be included. Short- and long-term goals and changes in the treatment program are often recorded here.

Plan: In this portion the therapist or assistant explains the treatment plan, recommended frequency of therapy, and prognosis if therapy is undertaken.

The following worksheet illustrates the information included in a SOAP note.

PHYSICAL THERAPY SOAP WORKSHEET

PATIENT'S NAME: JOHN H. DOE

SUBJECTIVE

Patient's complaint: John Doe is a 23-year-old man complaining of severe low back pain who was referred for physical therapy.

Nature of symptoms: Mr. Doe describes the pain as being a sharp, stabbing pain, which is constant and tingling all the way to the foot.

Location of symptoms: He says the pain begins in the left low back, moves to the left buttock, then runs down the front of the thigh, and goes to the big toe.

Behavior of symptoms: The pain is described as being worse in the morning and increasing drastically when the patient sits at a desk or bends forward. The pain is eased when the patient lies on his back with pillows under the knees or pulls the knees to the chest.

Onset of symptoms: Mr. Doe's pain began 2 days ago.

Course and duration of symptoms: There is no history of previous back injury or any other episodes of back pain. The day before the pain began, he spent the entire day putting away Christmas decorations in the attic.

Effect of previous treatment: He placed a heating pad on his back for 20-minute periods three times a day since his symptoms began with no relief. Mr. Doe also took Advil and Extra-Strength Tylenol with no relief.

Other related medical problems: The patient states he has had no weight loss, stomach problems, or history of malignancy.

OBJECTIVE

General observation: Mr. Doe is a well-nourished, 165-pound, 5'8" accountant who walks leaning to the left. He is very cooperative and anxious to receive treatment to decrease his symptoms because he has a business trip to New York City in 2 weeks.

Structural examination: On examination it is noted that the patient has an absence of lordosis, causing a flat appearance to the low back. He places his hands on his knees and pushes to stand.

Mobility examination: The patient has the following range of motion of the lumbar spine:

Flexion:	42 degrees
Extension:	15 degrees
Left rotation:	10 degrees
Right rotation:	20 degrees
Left lateral flexion:	12 degrees
Right lateral flexion:	15 degrees

Mr. Doe has pain at 45 degrees on the left with straight leg raising. His pain increases the most with forward flexion.

Neurological examination: The patient has a diminished knee reflex on the left. No muscle weakness is noted during manual muscle testing. Some numbness is noted in the L4 dermatome on the medial side of the leg and foot.

Palpation: Tenderness is noted on the left at L4-5. Severe muscle spasm is noted in the gluteal muscles on the left. The skin is not discolored, red, or hot.

Physician's report: X-ray films performed today in his doctor's office show mild narrowing of the disc space between the fourth and fifth lumbar vertebrae. He is to see the doctor again in 2 weeks at which time he will have an MRI if the symptoms have not improved.

Physical therapy treatment: After evaluation the patient received cold packs for 20 minutes, electric stimulation, and gentle massage. He was also instructed in proper body mechanics, home cold application, and gentle abdominal isometric exercises.

ASSESSMENT

Problem list: 1. Decreased range of motion of the spine
2. Increased muscle spasm and pain in the left low back area
3. Inability to work due to low sitting tolerance

Short-term goals: Decrease pain and muscle spasm in the low back area

Long-term goals: Increase spinal mobility to the normal range of motion
Decrease numbness and tingling in the left leg
Increase sitting tolerance

PLAN

Treatment: This patient will receive electrical stimulation, cold packs, massage, and abdominal isometric exercise, posture, and body mechanics instruction. He also will be instructed in a home program of self-stretches as his symptoms allow.

Frequency: Three times a day for 2 weeks

Prognosis: This patient appears to have a disc bulge at L4-5. The long-range prognosis will be determined after 2 weeks of acute treatment. If the patient's symptoms have subsided by at least 50% at that time, his prognosis will be good.

LEGAL AND ETHICAL ISSUES IN HEALTH CARE

The health care industry is regulated by both state and federal laws. Some of the laws that govern physical therapy originate from statutes passed by legislatures; other laws are derived from common law principles that have evolved from legal decisions.[3] As health care providers, physical therapy assistants must be familiar with laws associated with licensure, business, and employment. The risk of litigation can be minimized by regular review of legal implications of physical therapy practice. This section introduces some of the legal issues you may encounter as a physical therapy assistant.

Legal Concepts

Statutory laws

Laws that have an impact on physical therapy are statutory laws. These laws include licensure laws, workers' compensation law, Medicare/Medicaid, nondiscrimination laws (Rehabilitation Act of 1973, Civil Rights laws, Americans With Disabilities Act [ADA]), and tax code licensure laws applying to businesses.[3]

Liability

Defined as a duty that must be performed, liability can be a duty to carry out an act or a duty to abstain from doing something. To be liable means that an individual can be held accountable for harm caused to another individual. Harm that is the result of doing something is referred to as liability due to *commission* of a libelous act. Harm that is the result of failure to do something is referred to as liability due to *omission*. A claim of liability is the reason for most private lawsuits in the health care field.

Malpractice (negligence)

As citizens we are all liable for our actions. If harm is inflicted on another individual, the one injured may file a suit for compensation for the injury. This is referred to as a *negligence* suit. When an injury is implied in a suit against a medical professional, the term *malpractice* is used. Malpractice also is defined as the failure to exercise the training skills that normally would be exercised by other members of the profession with similar skills and training.

The following five factors are considered when deciding whether a health care professional is liable:

1. A duty was owed to the client.
2. There was a violation or breach of duty.
3. Harm resulted from the act or omission.
4. The act or omission was the cause of harm.
5. The harm was foreseeable.

Statute of limitations

Many different situations can result in allegations of professional carelessness. When a patient is injured or alleges injury, he or she can make a claim of medical malpractice within a specific time period. This legal time limit is known as the *statute of limitations*. In malpractice claims the statute of limitations is from 1 to 4 years because the passage of time makes gathering information difficult. This time begins from the time the damage is said to have occurred.

Risk management

Risk management is defined as the identification, analysis, and evaluation of risks and the selection of the most advantageous method for preventing them. The purposes of risk management programs are (1) to identify and eliminate potential situations that may lead to harm to employees, patients, or visitors and (2) to minimize the risk of civil suits.

Quality assurance (QA)

Quality assurance is defined by the Joint Commission on Accreditation of Hospitals (JCAH) as a "process designed to objectively and systematically monitor and evaluate the quality and appropriateness of patient care, pursue opportunities to improve patient care, and resolve identified problems." The JCAH along with the Professional Standards Review Organization (PSRO) are the agencies responsible for quality assurance.

Recommendations to Avoid Litigation

1. Conduct a thorough patient evaluation.
2. Seek consultation when in doubt.
3. Check the condition of departmental equipment.
4. Instruct patients thoroughly with written and oral instructions.
5. Keep the referring physician informed of patient's condition and progress.
6. Obtain proper consent for treatment.
7. Delegate only to qualified people.
8. Keep accurate, current, and well-written records.
9. Use a well-organized quality assurance program.

HEALTH INSURANCE

It is extremely important that all health care providers have a clear and thorough understanding of the policies and procedures of health insurance companies. There are four major classifications of health insurance and individual health plans: (1) private health insurance companies, (2) government health insurance, and (3) independent health plans, and (4) outcomes management systems.

During the last two or three decades, the one word that has come to describe our health care system is *change*. If physical therapists and physical therapist assistants are to function in this system, we must understand the historical events affecting it, which have brought about changes that affect us directly.

These changes have affected all four major classes of health insurance. The four classes are:

1. **Private Health Insurance Companies:** Included here are stock companies, mutual companies, and nonprofit insurance plans. Reimbursement for physical therapy is usually on a fee-for-service basis.
2. **Government Health Insurance:** Since the passage and implementation of Titles XVII (Medicare) and XIX (Medicaid) in 1965, the American health care system has undergone significant changes. The signing of Title XVIII of the Social Security Act in 1965 is considered to be the "most significant piece of health legislation ever passed by the U.S. Congress."[4] Medicaid, mandated by Title XIX of the Social Security Act, is a state-administered program intended to provide access to health care services for the poor, elderly, and disabled who do not receive coverage under Medicare.
3. **Independent Health Plans:** Health maintenance organizations (HMOs) and self-insurance plans are examples of independent health plans that are organized by various groups. Businesses, particularly large organizations, have sought to limit their financial risk through the use of HMOs, also referred to as managed care. Managed care organizations function as a link between providers and consumers. These organizations seek to control the utilization and cost of health care services.

4. **Outcomes Management Systems:** This type of health insurance is fairly new. Usually it involves gathering and analyzing the results of treatment and performances and then using the data to manage health care. These data come mainly from health care providers' billing, medical documentation, and reporting.[3]

According to one medical expert, the result of the movement to an outcomes management system is that purchasers and providers of health care are looking for treatment programs designed and based on "outcomes that are known to aid patients in returning to normal function, both medically and socially in the shortest period of time."[5]

GUIDELINES FOR CONDUCT OF THE AFFILIATE MEMBER OF THE AMERICAN PHYSICAL THERAPY ASSOCIATION (APTA)

This guide is a reference for physical therapist assistants in the interpretation of the "Standards of Ethical Conduct for the Physical Therapist Assistant," written by the American Physical Therapy Association.[6]

Standard 1

Physical therapist assistants provide services under the supervision of a physical therapist.

1.1 Supervisory relationships

Physical therapist assistants shall work under the supervision and direction of a physical therapist who is properly credentialed in the jurisdiction in which the physical therapist assistant practices.

1.2 Performance of service

A. Physical therapist assistants may not initiate or alter a treatment program without prior evaluation by and approval of the supervising physical therapist.
B. Physical therapist assistants may, with prior approval by the supervising physical therapist, adjust a specific treatment procedure in accordance with changes in patient status.
C. Physical therapist assistants may not interpret data beyond the scope of their physical therapist assistant education.
D. Physical therapist assistants may respond to inquiries regarding patient status to appropriate parties within the protocol established by a supervising physical therapist.
E. Physical therapist assistants shall refer inquiries regarding patient prognosis to a supervising physical therapist.

Standard 2

Physical therapist assistants respect the rights and dignity of all individuals.

2.1 Attitudes of physical therapist assistants

A. Physical therapist assistants shall recognize that each individual is different from all other individuals and respect and be responsive to those differences.
B. Physical therapist assistants shall be guided at all times by concern for the dignity and welfare of those patients entrusted to their care.
C. Physical therapist assistants shall be responsive to and supportive of colleagues and associates.

2.2 Request for release of information

Physical therapist assistants shall refer all requests for release of confidential information to the supervising physical therapist.

2.3 Protection of privacy

Physical therapist assistants must treat as confidential all information relating to the personal conditions and affairs of the persons whom they serve.

Standard 3

Physical therapist assistants maintain and promote high standards in the provisions of services, giving the welfare of patients their highest regard.

3.1 Information about services

Physical therapist assistants may provide consumers with information regarding provision of services within the protocol established by a supervising physical therapist.

Physical therapist assistants may not use, or participate in the use of, any form of communication containing a false, fraudulent, misleading, deceptive, unfair, or sensational statement or claim.

3.2 Organizational employment

Physical therapist assistants shall advise their employer(s) of any employer practice that causes them to be in conflict with the "Standards of Ethical Conduct for the Physical Therapist Assistant."

3.3 Endorsement of equipment

Physical therapist assistants may not endorse equipment or exercise influence on patients or families to purchase or lease equipment except as directed by a physical therapist acting in accord with the stipulation in paragraph 5.3A of the *Guide for Conduct of the Affiliate Member.*[5]

3.4 Financial considerations

Physical therapist assistants shall never place their own financial interest above the welfare of their patients.

3.5 Exploitation of patients

Physical therapist assistants shall not participate in any arrangements in which patients are exploited. Such arrangements include situations in which referring sources enhance their personal incomes as a result of referring for, delegating, prescribing, or recommending physical therapy services.

Standard 4

Physical therapist assistants provide services within the limits of the law.

4.1 Supervisory relationships

Physical therapist assistants shall comply with all aspects of law. Regardless of the content of any law, physical therapist assistants shall provide services only under the supervision and direction of a physical therapist who is properly credentialed in the jurisdiction in which the physical therapist assistant practices.

4.2 Representation

Physical therapist assistants shall not falsely present themselves as physical therapists.

Standard 5

Physical therapist assistants make those judgments that are commensurate with their qualifications as physical therapist assistants.

5.1 Patient treatment

Physical therapist assistants shall report all untoward patient responses to a supervising physical therapist.

5.2 Patient safety

Physical therapist assistants may refuse to carry out treatment procedures that they believe are not in the best interest of the patient.

5.3 Qualifications

Physical therapist assistants may not carry out any procedure that they are not qualified to provide.

5.4 Discontinuance of treatment program

Physical therapist assistants shall discontinue immediately any treatment procedures that in their judgment appear to be harmful to the patient.

5.5 Continued education

Physical therapist assistants shall continue participation in various types of educational activities that enhance their skills and knowledge and provide new skills and knowledge.

Standard 6

Physical therapist assistants give the welfare of patients their highest regard.

6.1 Financial consideration

Physical therapist assistants shall never place their own financial interest above the welfare of their patients.

6.2 Exploitation of patients

Physical therapist assistants shall not participate in any arrangements in which patients are exploited. Such arrangements include situations in which referring sources enhance their personal incomes as a result of referring for, delegating, prescribing, or recommending physical therapy services.

REVIEW QUESTIONS

1. When the physical therapist or physical therapist assistant writes a progress note, he or she may use a SOAP note. What does the "A" stand for?
   a. Activity
   b. Assessment
   c. Action
   d. Acute symptoms
2. A physical therapist assistant would be incorrect if he or she placed which of the following information in the assessment section of a SOAP note?
   a. "Patient should be independent with crutches on discharge"
   b. "Left quadriceps strength is within normal limits"
   c. "Patient continues to make steady progress with upper extremity exercises"
   d. "EMG shows nerve damage"
3. It is important for physical therapists to be familiar with the educational background, standards of practice, and current issues affecting physical therapist assistants. Which of the following is *not* accurate?
   a. Physical therapist assistants may be affiliate members of the APTA
   b. Physical therapist assistants are regulated in all 50 states
   c. It is cost-effective to employ physical therapist assistants
   d. Career advancement for the physical therapist assistant may be limited in many facilities
4. In a SOAP note the "S" stands for subjective data. Which of the following is classified as subjective information?
   a. Physical examination
   b. Diagnosis
   c. Prescribed treatment and progress note
   d. Patient's family history
5. "SOAP" is an acronym that refers to:
   a. Medical records
   b. Malpractice
   c. Dictation equipment
   d. Telephone equipment
6. The POMR is also called the:
   a. SOAP system
   b. Source-related system
   c. Weed system
   d. System-related record
7. The SOAP type of progress notes are:
   a. Problem solving
   b. Unstructured
   c. Too long
   d. Uncommon form of note writing

8. What does the acronym "POMR" stand for?
   a. Physical/occupational medicine record
   b. Performance objective medical record
   c. Problem-oriented medical record
   d. Preferred-oriented medical record

9. In the SOAP format, the physical therapist assistant would place the short-term goals for a patient in which section?
   a. Subjective
   b. Objective
   c. Assessment
   d. Plan

10. In the SOAP note, the short-term goals should be stated:
    a. After the long-term goals
    b. Before the long-term goals
    c. At the same time as the long-term goals
    d. It doesn't matter

11. In a problem-oriented medical record, a physical therapist assistant writes, "patient complained of pain in back when sitting." In which section of the SOAP note should this information be placed?
    a. Subjective
    b. Plan
    c. Assessment
    d. Objective

12. What do the letters "DRG" stand for?
    a. Diagnostic-ruled groups
    b. Diagnostic-related groups
    c. Disease-related groups
    d. Diagnostic-related generation

13. Patient documentation is important and necessary for:
    a. Communication with other staff members
    b. Legal implications
    c. Quality assurance
    d. Research
    e. All of the above

14. When the physical therapist assistant uses the SOAP format, the "S" stands for:
    a. Symptoms
    b. Signs
    c. Subjective
    d. Social history

15. The order in which progress notes, x-ray films, and laboratory work are added to the patient's record is:
    a. Subjective
    b. Objective
    c. Chronological
    d. Problem oriented

16. The system of medical records developed by Lawrence Weed is called:
    a. POMR
    b. MCRI
    c. DRG
    d. ADPR

17. Patients may qualify for Medicaid depending on:
    a. Amount of Social Security they receive
    b. Other insurance enrolled in
    c. Their income
    d. Nature of illness
18. HMO stands for:
    a. Health management objective
    b. Health maintenance organization
    c. Health membership organization
    d. Health measurement organization
19. A physical therapist assistant is working without a physical therapist in the clinic for 3 days. The assistant can do all the following *except:*
    a. Supervise rehabilitation exercises
    b. Modify treatment plan
    c. Gait training
    d. Write progress notes
20. Health maintenance organizations are a growing and popular type of insurance provider. They are most likely to limit physical therapy coverage based on:
    a. Duration of each physical therapy treatment
    b. Number of modalities
    c. Number of visits
    d. Frequency of visits
21. A physical therapist assistant should chart observed information on range of motion in which section of the SOAP note?
    a. Subjective
    b. Objective
    c. Assessment
    d. Plan
22. The role of the physical therapist assistant may vary from clinic to clinic. Which of the following duties generally should *not* be performed by the assistant?
    a. Crutch ambulation
    b. Hot packs and ice packs
    c. Ultrasound
    d. Initial evaluations
23. Which of the following would *not* be found in the objective section of a SOAP note?
    a. Range of motion measurements
    b. Description of present treatment
    c. Vital signs
    d. Long-term goals
24. The physical therapist assistant should record his or her professional judgment in which section of a SOAP note?
    a. Subjective
    b. Objective
    c. Assessment
    d. Plan

25. Which of the following would help to protect you against a lawsuit?
    a. Recording of accurate and regular progress notes
    b. Constantly supervising all patient activities
    c. Increasing malpractice insurance
    d. All of the above
26. You are a physical therapist assistant in a large clinic and are working in the gym area. You observe a patient who, 10 weeks following anterior cruciate ligament surgery, is performing his exercises without any effort. You should:
    a. Call the doctor and tell him or her that the physical therapist needs to reevaluate the patient
    b. Do nothing until the physical therapist notices the need to increase the patient's workout
    c. Alter the patient's program as you think necessary
    d. Consult your supervising physical therapist and give your recommended treatment changes
27. You answer the phone in a physical therapy clinic, and an attorney asks for medical information on an individual whom she says is receiving physical therapy for a fractured patella. You should:
    a. Pull the chart and give her the requested information
    b. Inform the attorney that you are too busy to assist her
    c. Tell the attorney to get the appropriate forms signed and then she can call you back to discuss the patient's situation
    d. Instruct the attorney to get the appropriate forms signed and you will send the patient's records to the appropriate person

REFERENCES
1. Stewart DL, Abeln SH: *Documenting functional outcomes in physical therapy,* St Louis, 1993, Mosby.
2. Nosse LJ, Friberg DG: *Management principles for physical therapists,* Baltimore, 1992, Williams & Wilkins.
3. Walter J: *Physical therapy management: an integrated science,* St Louis, 1993, Mosby.
4. Reinecker P: Catholic health care enters a new world, *Health Prog,* June, pp 31-36, 1990.
5. Hubbard DD: Views, *Healthweek,* pp 94-96, August 12, 1991.
6. The Judicial Committee: *Guide for conduct of the affiliate member,* Alexandria, Va, 1991, American Physical Therapy Association.

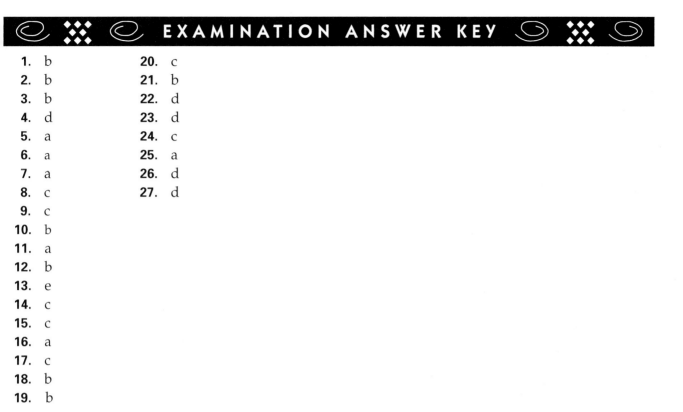

EXAMINATION ANSWER KEY

1. b	**20.** c		
2. b	**21.** b		
3. b	**22.** d		
4. d	**23.** d		
5. a	**24.** c		
6. a	**25.** a		
7. a	**26.** d		
8. c	**27.** d		
9. c			
10. b			
11. a			
12. b			
13. e			
14. c			
15. c			
16. a			
17. c			
18. b			
19. b			

EXAMINATION ANSWER SHEET

1. _____   21. _____

2. _____   22. _____

3. _____   23. _____

4. _____   24. _____

5. _____   25. _____

6. _____   26. _____

7. _____   27. _____

8. _____

9. _____

10. _____

11. _____

12. _____

13. _____

14. _____

15. _____

16. _____

17. _____

18. _____

19. _____

20. _____

EXAMINATION ANSWER SHEET

1. _____   21. _____

2. _____   22. _____

3. _____   23. _____

4. _____   24. _____

5. _____   25. _____

6. _____   26. _____

7. _____   27. _____

8. _____

9. _____

10. _____

11. _____

12. _____

13. _____

14. _____

15. _____

16. _____

17. _____

18. _____

19. _____

20. _____

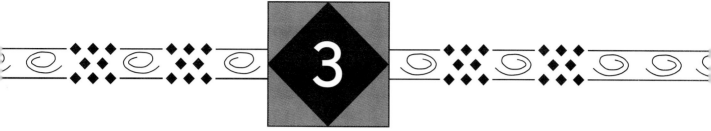

Anatomy, Physiology, Kinesiology

This chapter reviews the structure, function, and movement of the human body as it relates to the practice of physical therapy. For this reason the subjects of anatomy, physiology, and kinesiology have been grouped together. By definition, *anatomy* is the study of the structure of the human body, *physiology* is the study of the function of the human body, and *kinesiology* is the study of movement of the human body. This chapter emphasizes the muscular, skeletal, cardiovascular, respiratory, and nervous systems.

An understanding of these subjects is prerequisite to being able to apply even the most basic principles and procedures related to your physical therapy skills. A solid knowledge of the normal structure and function of the human body provides the necessary foundation to be able to recognize specific clinical conditions seen and treated in the physical therapy clinic.

TERMINOLOGY

When beginning the study and review of anatomy, physiology, and kinesiology, you may find the number of medical terms overwhelming. However, it is extremely important to use correct terminology when writing reports or talking with colleagues to avoid confusion and mistakes.

Chapter 1 focused on prefixes, suffixes, and root words. This section emphasizes words that relate specifically to anatomy, physiology, and kinesiology.

Terms	Definitions
For terms 1-14, see Figs. 3-1 and 3-2.	
1. Left	Toward left side
2. Right	Toward right side
3. Superior	Above or higher than another structure
4. Inferior	Below or lower than another structure
5. Cephalic	Closer to head
6. Caudal	Closer to tail or feet
7. Proximal	Closer to trunk
8. Distal	Away from trunk
9. Medial	Toward midline
10. Lateral	Away from midline
11. Anterior	Toward front
12. Posterior	Toward back
13. Ventral	Toward belly (anterior)
14. Dorsal	Toward back (posterior)

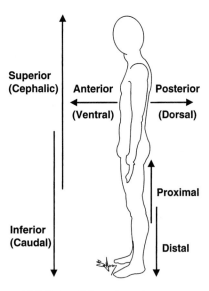

FIG 3-1. Directional terms.

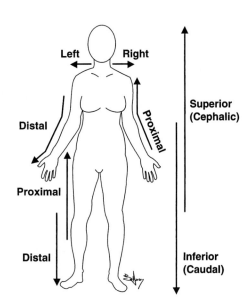

FIG 3-2. Directional terms.

Terms	Definitions
15. Superficial	Toward surface
16. Deep	Away from surface
17. Biomechanics	Mechanical principles related to body
18. Static	Nonmoving
19. Dynamic	Moving
20. Kinetics	Forces that cause movement
21. Kinematics	Time, space, and mass aspect of motion
22. Fundamental position	Position in which person is standing with feet facing forward, arms at sides, palms facing side of body (Fig. 3-3)
23. Anatomical position	Same as fundamental position but palms face forward (Fig. 3-4)
24. Linear motion (translatory)	Motion occurring in more or less a straight line; movement occurs at same distance, same direction, and same time
25. Rectilinear motion	Linear motion in straight line
26. Curvilinear motion	Linear motion in straight line but curved path
27. Angular motion (rotary)	Motion in which parts move through same angle and direction at same time but not for same distance
28. Flexion	Bending movement (decrease angle) (Fig. 3-5)
29. Extension	Straightening movement (increase angle) (Fig. 3-6)
30. Abduction	Movement away from midline (Fig. 3-7)
31. Adduction	Movement toward midline (Fig. 3-7)
32. Circumduction	Combination of flexion, extension, abduction, and adduction
33. Internal rotation (medial)	Movement of anterior surface toward midline (Fig. 3-8)
34. External rotation (lateral)	Movement of anterior surface away from midline (Fig. 3-9)
35. Inversion	Turning sole of foot inward at ankle (Fig. 3-10)
36. Eversion	Turning sole of foot outward at ankle (Fig. 3-11)
37. Protraction	Movement anterior/away from midline (abduction)
38. Retraction	Movement posterior/toward midline (adduction)
39. Supination	Rotation of palm so that it faces anteriorly (Fig. 3-12)
40. Pronation	Rotation of palm so that it faces posteriorly (Fig. 3-13)
41. Palmar flexion	Flexion at wrist (Fig. 3-14)
42. Plantar flexion	Movement of foot toward plantar surface (Fig. 3-15)
43. Dorsiflexion	Ankle—movement of foot toward shin Wrist—movement of dorsum of hand posteriorly (Fig. 3-15)

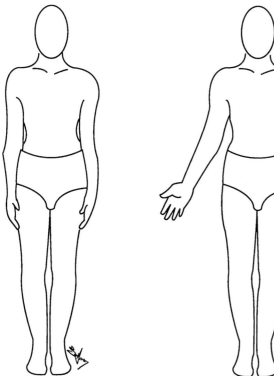

FIG 3-3.   Fundamental position.

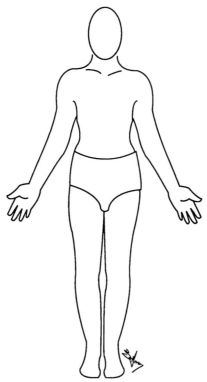

FIG 3-4.   Anatomical position.

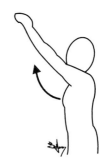

FIG 3-5.   Shoulder flexion.

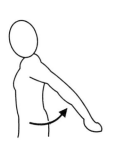

FIG 3-6.   Shoulder extension.

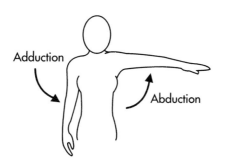

FIG 3-7.   Shoulder abduction.

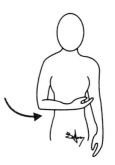

FIG 3-8.   Shoulder internal rotation.

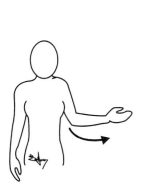

FIG 3-9.   Shoulder external rotation.

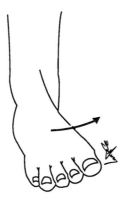

FIG 3-10.   Ankle inversion.

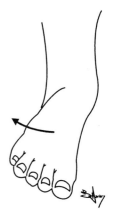

FIG 3-11.   Ankle eversion.

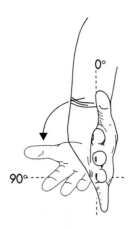

FIG 3-12

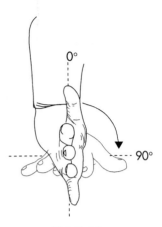

FIG 3-13

FIG 3-12. Radioulnar supination. (From Hartley A: *Practical joint assessment: upper quadrant,* ed 2, St Louis, 1995, Mosby.)

FIG 3-13. Radioulnar pronation. (From Hartley A: *Practical joint assessment: upper quadrant,* ed 2, St Louis, 1995, Mosby.)

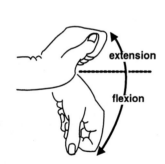

FIG 3-14. Palmar flexion.

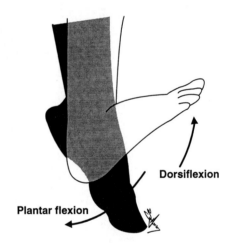

FIG 3-15. Ankle plantar flexion/dorsiflexion.

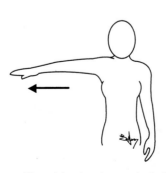

FIG 3-16. Shoulder horizontal abduction.

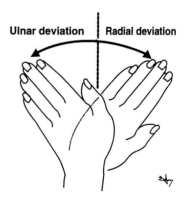

FIG 3-17. Ulnar/radial deviation.

Terms	**Definitions**
44. Horizontal abduction	Movement in which shoulder is flexed to 90 degrees and then abducted (Fig. 3-16)
45. Horizontal adduction	Movement in which shoulder is flexed to 90 degrees and then adducted
46. Ulnar deviation	Movement of hand medially from anatomical position toward ulnar side of wrist (Fig. 3-17)
47. Radial deviation	Movement of hand laterally from anatomical position toward radial side of wrist (Fig. 3-17)
48. Lateral flexion	Movement of trunk sideways
49. Axial skeleton	Bones of skull, hyoid, vertebral column, and rib cage (Fig. 3-18)
50. Appendicular skeleton	Bones of limbs and their girdles (Fig. 3-19)

For terms 51-58, see Fig. 3-20

51. Compact bone	Hard, dense outer shell of bone
52. Cancellous (spongy) bone	Porous, spongy inside part of bone
53. Diaphysis	Shaft of bone
54. Epiphysis	End of bone
55. Periosteum	Connective tissue membrane covering outer surface of bone except where articular cartilage is present
56. Endosteum	Tissue lining inner cavities of bone
57. Articular cartilage	Thin layer of hyaline cartilage covering bone where it forms bone
58. Medullary cavity	Large cavity within diaphysis
59. Osteoblast	Cell that produces bone matrix
60. Osteocyte	Bone cell surrounded by bone matrix
61. Red marrow	Site of blood cell production
62. Yellow marrow	Fat stored within medullary cavity
63. Long bone	Tubular-shaped bone in which its length is greater than its width
64. Short bone	Cubical-shaped bone
65. Flat bone	Thin, curved bone consisting of two layers of cancellous bone
66. Sesamoid bone	Oval-shaped bone found within tendons
67. Body	Main portion of a bone

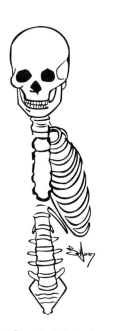

FIG 3-18. Axial skeleton.

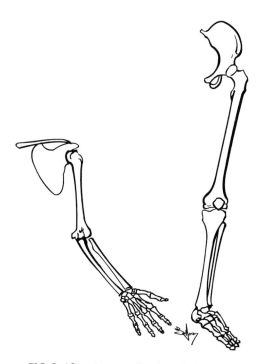

FIG 3-19. Appendicular skeleton.

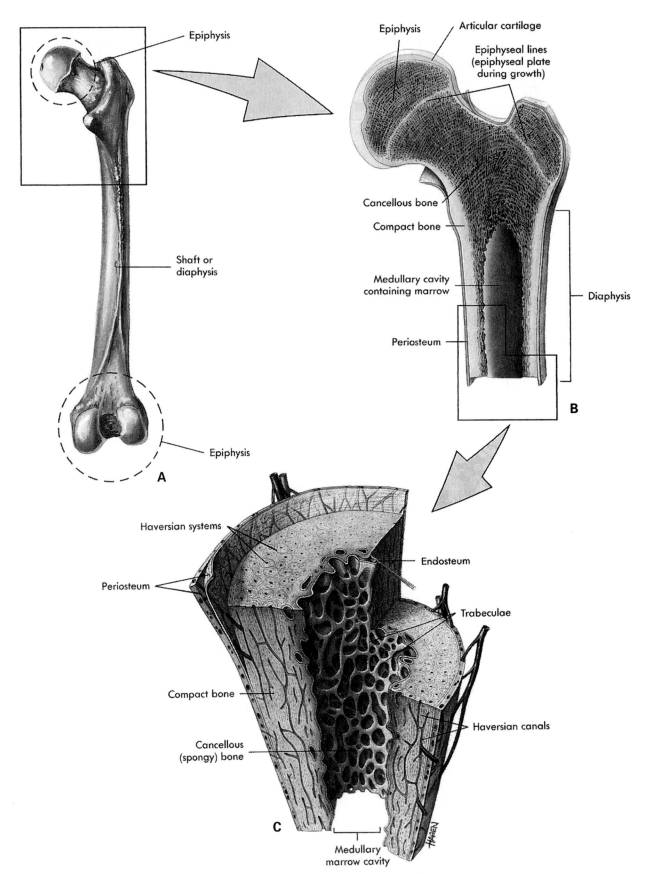

FIG 3-20.   A, Young long bone (femur) showing epiphyses, epiphyseal plates, and diaphysis. **B,** Adult long bone with epiphyseal lines. **C,** Internal features of a portion of the long bone in **B.** (Courtesy John V. Hagen.)

Terms	Definitions
68. Head	Enlarged, rounded end of a bone
69. Neck	Constricted area of a bone between its head and neck
70. Ramus	Branch off the body of a bone
71. Condyle	Smooth, rounded articular surface
72. Facet	Small, flattened articular surface
73. Linea (line)	Low ridge
74. Crest	Prominent ridge
75. Spine	Very high ridge
76. Tubercle	Small, rounded process
77. Tuberosity	Large, rounded process
78. Trochanter	Large tuberosity on proximal femur
79. Epicondyle	Near or above a condyle
80. Foramen	Hole or opening through which blood vessels, nerves, or ligaments pass
81. Fossa	Depression
82. Sinus	Air-filled cavity in a bone
83. Meatus	Canal in a bone
84. Fibrous joint (synarthrosis)	Joint in which two bones are united by fibrous tissue (Fig. 3-21)
85. Cartilaginous joint (amphiarthrosis)	Joint in which two bones are united by either hyaline cartilage or fibrocartilage (Fig. 3-22)

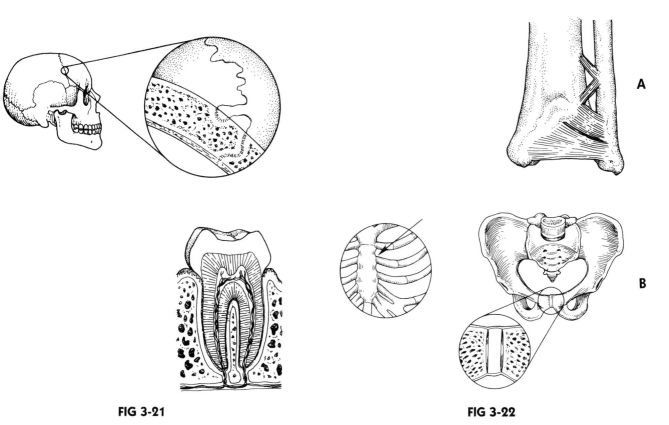

FIG 3-21.   **FIG 3-22.**

FIG 3-21.   Synarthrodial joints. (From Thompson CW, Floyd RT: *Manual of structural kinesiology,* ed 12, St Louis, 1994, Mosby.

FIG 3-22.   Amphiarthrodial joints. **A,** Syndesmosis joint. **B,** Synchondrosis joint. (From Thompson CW, Floyd RT: *Manual of structural kinesiology,* ed 12, St Louis, 1994, Mosby.)

Terms	Definitions
86. Synovial joint diarthrosis)	Joint with no direct union between the two bones; joint cavity is filled with fluid (Fig. 3-23)
87. Nonaxial joint	Joint in which only gliding motion is possible
88. Uniaxial joint	Joint that has one axis and allows movement in one plane (flexion-extension-sagittal plane)
89. Biaxial joint	Joint that has two axes and allows movement in two planes (flexion-extension-sagittal plane, abduction-adduction-frontal plane)
90. Triaxial joint	Joint that has three axes and allows movement in three planes (flexion-extension-sagittal plane, abduction-adduction-frontal plane, rotation-transverse plane)
91. Hyaline cartilage (articular)	Cartilage that covers the ends of opposing bones
92. Fibrocartilage	Cartilage that acts as a shock absorber between opposing bones
93. Labrum	Ring of fibrocartilage around shoulder and hip joints that increases depth of joint cavity
94. Aponeurosis	Tendinous sheet in which tendons attach to bones
95. Linea alba	Aponeurosis attachment of the abdominal muscles at the midline
96. Bursa	Padlike sac under tendons
97. Origin	Fixed attachment of muscle
98. Insertion	Place of attachment of a muscle to the bone that it moves
99. Reversal of muscle action	Movement in which muscle origin moves toward insertion
100. Strap muscle	Long, thin fibers that run length of muscle

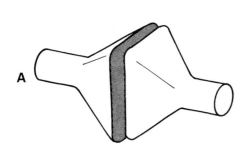
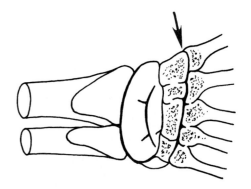
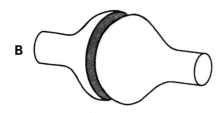
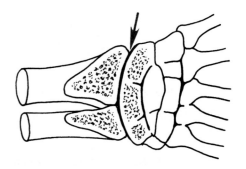

FIG 3-23. Diarthrodial joints. **A,** Arthrodial joint. **B,** Condyloidal joint.

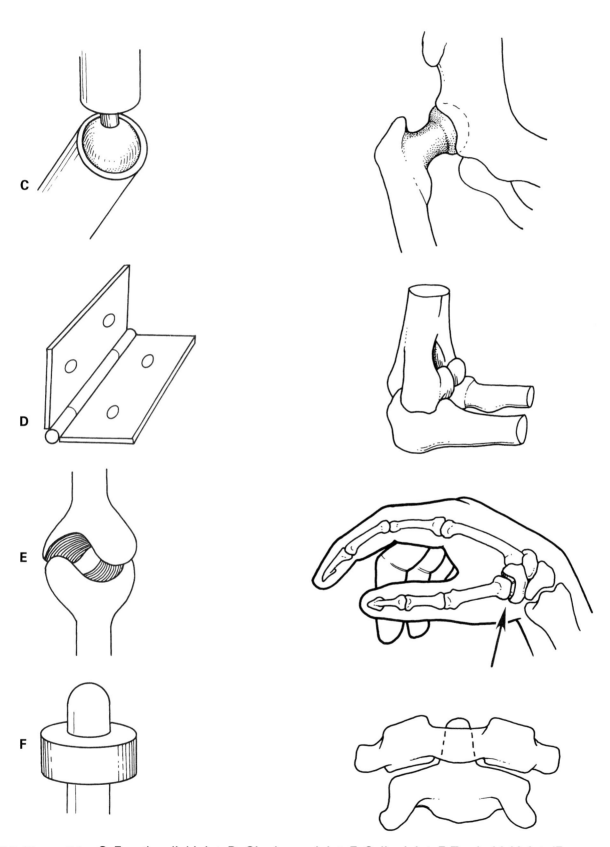

FIG 3-23, cont'd.   **C,** Enarthrodial joint. **D,** Ginglymus joint. **E,** Sellar joint. **F,** Trochoidal joint. (From
Thompson CW, Floyd RT: *Manual of structural kinesiology,* ed 12, St Louis, 1994, Mosby.)

FIG 3-24.   Examples of muscle shapes. **A,** Unipennate. **B,** Bipennate. **C,** Multipennate (triangular). **D,** Quadrate. **E,** Trapezoid. **F,** Rhomboid. **G,** Fusiform. **H,** Digastric. **I,** Bicipital. (Courtesy John V. Hagen.)

Terms	Definitions
For terms 101-106, see Fig. 3-24)	
101. Fusiform muscle	Spindle-shaped muscle that is wider in middle and has tendons on both ends
102. Rhomboid muscle	Flat, four-sided muscle with broad attachments
103. Triangular muscle	Flat, fan-shaped muscle with narrow attachment at one end and broad attachment at the other
104. Unipennate muscle	Muscle with fasciculi (fibers) on one side of central tendon
105. Bipennate muscle	Muscle with fasciculi on both sides of central tendon
106. Multipennate muscle	Muscle with many tendons and fibers in between
107. Irritability	Ability to respond to a stimulus
108. Contractility	Ability to shorten or contract (produce tension)
109. Extensibility	Ability to stretch or lengthen when force is applied
110. Elasticity	Ability to recoil or return to resting length
111. Tension	Force built up in a muscle
112. Active insufficiency	Inability of a muscle to act (shorten)
113. Passive insufficiency	Inability of muscle to lengthen any farther without injury
114. Tenodesis	Tendon action of a muscle (stretch)
115. Synergist	Muscle that works together with another muscle to cause movement
116. Neutralizer	Prevents unwanted motion
117. Agonist (prime mover)	Muscle that causes motion
118. Antagonist	Muscle whose action is opposite of that of agonist
119. Stabilizer	Muscle that supports and allows agonist to work
120. Isometric contraction	Muscle contraction in which muscle produces constant tension and muscle length remains the same
121. Isotonic contraction	Muscle contraction in which muscle produces constant tension and muscle shortens or lengthens
122. Isokinetic contraction	Muscle contraction in which muscle shortens at constant speed and tension is maximal over full range of motion
123. Concentric contraction	Muscle contraction in which muscle contracts and muscle attachments move toward each other
124. Eccentric contraction	Lengthening muscle contraction in which muscle attachments separate

MUSCULAR SYSTEM

Muscle tissue is specialized and is responsible for the movement and positioning of the skeletal segments of the body. There are three types of muscle tissue: skeletal, cardiac, and smooth. Skeletal muscle moves the trunk and extremities, cardiac muscle propels blood through vessels, and smooth muscle forces food through the digestive system.[1] This section presents the basic structure and function of muscle tissue, with emphasis on skeletal muscle.

Muscle Action by Joint
Temporomandibular joint

Depression	Elevation	Protraction	Side to side
Pterygoid lateralis	Temporalis	Masseter	Temporalis of same side
Suprahyoid	Masseter	Pterygoid lateralis	Pterygoid of opposite side
Infrahyoid	Pterygoid medialis	Pterygoid medialis	Masseter

Cervical joints

Flexion	Extension	Rotation and lateral flexion
Sternocleidomastoid	Splenius capitis	Scalene muscles
Longus colli	Splenius cervicis	Splenius capitis
Longus capitis	Semispinalis cervicis	Splenius cervicis
	Iliocostalis cervicis	Longissimus capitis
	Longissimus capitis	Longissimus cervicis
		Multifidus muscles

Thoracic and lumbar joints

Flexion	Extension	Rotation and lateral flexion
Rectus abdominis	Erector spinae	Psoas major
	Quadratus lumborum	Quadratus lumborum
		External oblique
		Internal oblique
		Multifidus muscles
		Iliocostalis lumborum
		Iliocostalis thoracis
		Rotatores muscles

Scapula

Elevation	Depression	Protraction	Retraction	Superior rotation	Inferior rotation
Trapezius	Pectoralis minor	Pectoralis minor	Trapezius	Trapezius	Levator scapulae
Levator scapulae	Latissimus dorsi	Serratus anterior	Rhomboid muscles	Serratus anterior	Rhomboid muscles
					Pectoralis minor

Shoulder joint

Flexion	Extension	Abduction	Adduction	External rotation	Internal rotation
Pectoralis major	Latissimus dorsi	Deltoid (middle)	Pectoralis major	Deltoid	Pectoralis major
Deltoid (anterior)	Deltoid (posterior)	Supraspinatus	Latissimus dorsi	Teres minor	Latissimus dorsi
Coracobrachialis	Teres major			Infraspinatus	Teres major
Biceps brachii	Pectoralis major				Subscapularis
					Deltoid

Elbow joint

Flexion	Extension
Brachialis	Triceps
Biceps brachii	Anconeus
Brachioradialis	

Radioulnar joint

Supination	Pronation
Supinator	Pronator quadratus
Biceps brachii	Pronator teres

Wrist joint

Flexion	Extension	Radial deviation	Ulnar deviation
Flexor carpi radialis	Extensor carpi radialis longus	Extensor carpi radialis longus	Flexor carpi ulnaris
Flexor carpi ulnaris	Extensor carpi radialis brevis	Extensor carpi radialis brevis	Extensor carpi ulnaris
Palmaris longus	Extensor carpi ulnaris	Flexor carpi radialis	
		Abductor pollicis longus	

Hip joint

Flexion	Extension	Abduction	Adduction	Internal rotation	External rotation
Iliopsoas	Gluteus maximus	Gluteus medius	Adductor magnus	Tensor fasciae	Obturator internus
Tensor fasciae	Semitendinosus	Gluteus minimus	Adductor longus	Gluteus medius	Obturator externus
Rectus femoris	Semimembranosus		Adductor brevis	Gluteus minimus	Piriformis
	Biceps femoris				Quadriceps femoris
					Gemellus muscles

Knee joint

Flexion	Extension	Internal rotation of flexed leg	Lateral rotation of flexed leg
Semimembranosus	Rectus femoris	Popliteus	Biceps femoris
Semitendinosus	Vastus lateralis	Semitendinosus	
Biceps femoris	Vastus intermedius	Semimembranosus	
	Vastus medialis		

Ankle joint

Dorsiflexion	Plantar flexion
Tibialis anterior	Gastrocnemius
Extensor hallucis longus	Soleus
	Peroneus longus

Subtalar joint

Inversion	Eversion	Plantar flexion
Tibialis anterior	Peroneus longus	Peroneus longus
Tibialis posterior	Peroneus brevis	Tibialis posterior
	Peroneus tertius	Abductor hallucis
		Abductor digiti minimi
		Flexor digitorum brevis

Major Muscles of the Extremities—Origins and Insertions

When you are learning the origins and insertions of the various muscles in the body, the process should include studying charts of origins and insertions, visualizing and locating the origins and insertions on a skeleton, studying illustrations of each muscle, and when possible palpating the muscle on yourself or a lab partner. Figs. 3-25 through 3-94 illustrate the origins, insertions, and actions of the major skeletal muscles in the body.

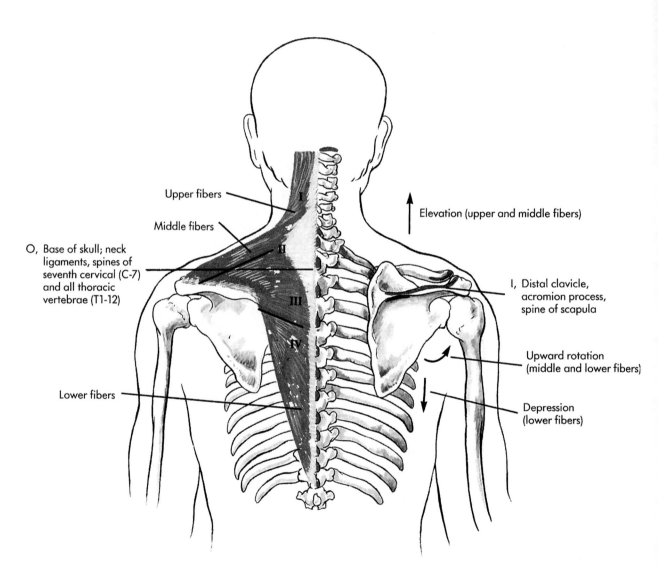

FIG 3-25.   Trapezius muscle. *O,* Origin; *I,* insertion.   (From Thompson CW, Floyd RT: *Manual of structural kinesiology,* ed 12, St Louis, 1994, Mosby.)

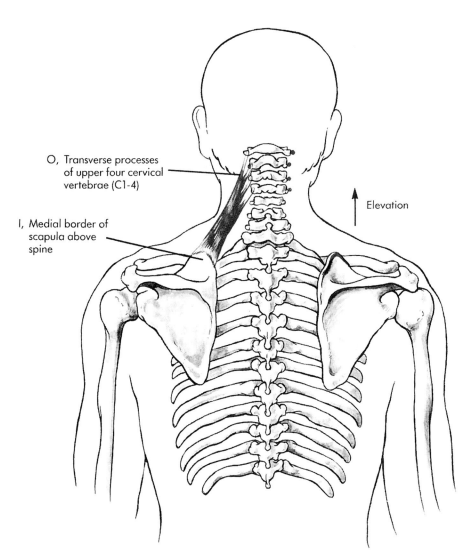

O, Transverse processes
of upper four cervical
vertebrae (C1-4)

I, Medial border of
scapula above
spine

Elevation

FIG 3-26. Levator scapulae muscle. *O,* Origin; *I,* insertion. (From Thompson CW, Floyd RT: *Manual of structural kinesiology,* ed 12, St Louis, 1994, Mosby.)

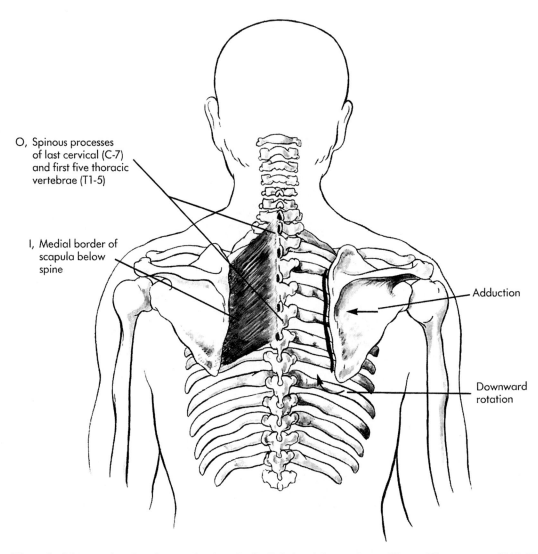

O, Spinous processes
of last cervical (C-7)
and first five thoracic
vertebrae (T1-5)

I, Medial border of
scapula below
spine

Adduction

Downward
rotation

FIG 3-27. Rhomboid muscles (major and minor). *O,* Origin; *I,* insertion. (From Thompson CW, Floyd RT: *Manual of structural kinesiology,* ed 12, St Louis, 1994, Mosby.)

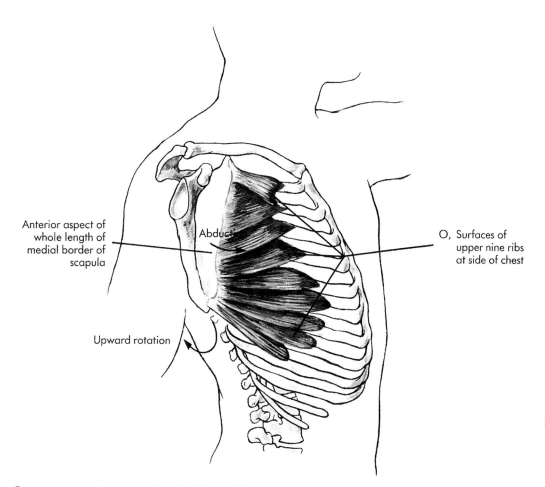

Anterior aspect of
whole length of
medial border of
scapula

Abduct

Upward rotation

O, Surfaces of
upper nine ribs
at side of chest

FIG 3-28.   Serratus anterior muscle. *O,* Origin; *I,* insertion. (From Thompson CW, Floyd RT: *Manual of structural kinesiology,* ed 12, St Louis, 1994, Mosby.)

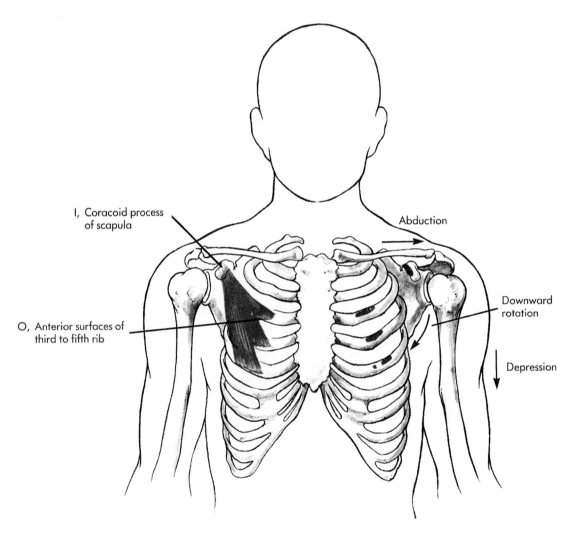

I, Coracoid process
of scapula

Abduction

O, Anterior surfaces of
third to fifth rib

Downward
rotation

Depression

FIG 3-29.   Pectoralis minor muscle. *O,* Origin; *I,* insertion. (From Thompson CW, Floyd RT: *Manual of structural kinesiology,* ed 12, St Louis, 1994, Mosby.)

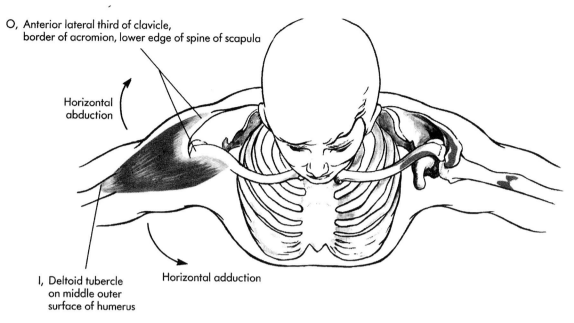

O, Anterior lateral third of clavicle,
border of acromion, lower edge of spine of scapula

Horizontal
abduction

I, Deltoid tubercle
on middle outer
surface of humerus

Horizontal adduction

IG 3-30.   Deltoid muscle. *O,* Origin; *I,* insertion. (From Thompson CW, Floyd RT: *Manual of structural kinesiology,* ed 12, St Louis, 1994, Mosby.)

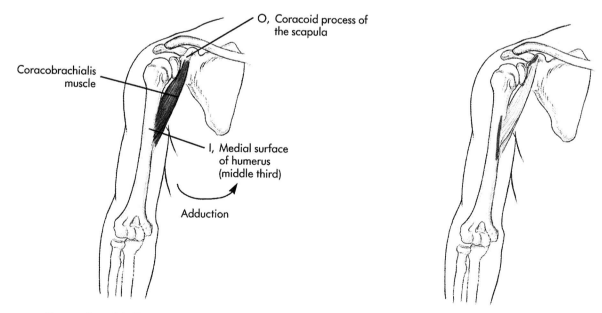

O, Coracoid process of
the scapula

Coracobrachialis
muscle

I, Medial surface
of humerus
(middle third)

Adduction

IG 3-31.   Coracobrachialis muscle. *O,* Origin; *I,* insertion. (From Thompson CW, Floyd RT: *Manual of structural kinesiology,* ed 12, St Louis, 1994, Mosby.)

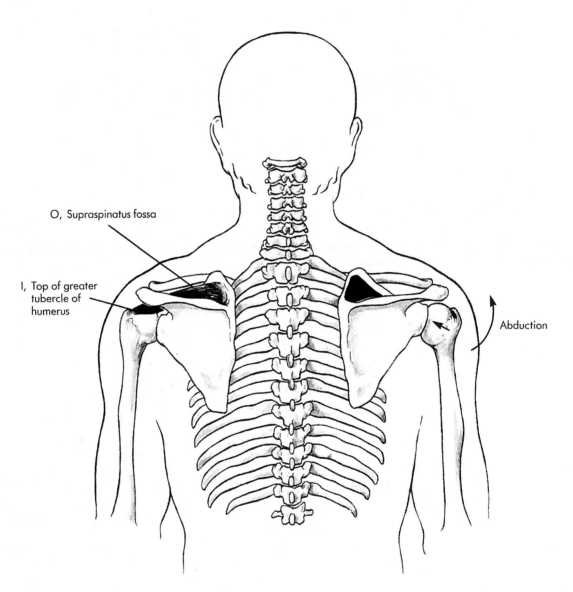

O, Supraspinatus fossa

I, Top of greater
tubercle of
humerus

Abduction

FIG 3-32.   Supraspinatus muscle. *O,* Origin; *I,* insertion. (From Thompson CW, Floyd RT: *Manual of structural kinesiology,* ed 12, St Louis, 1994, Mosby.)

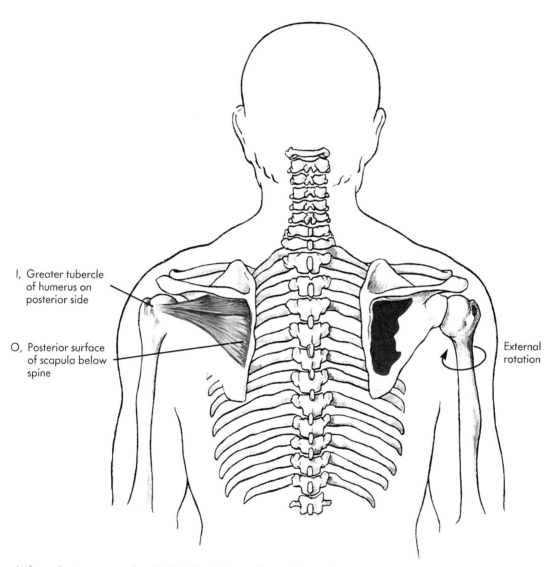

I, Greater tubercle
of humerus on
posterior side

O, Posterior surface
of scapula below
spine

External
rotation

FIG 3-33.   Infraspinatus muscle. *O,* Origin; *I,* insertion. (From Thompson CW, Floyd RT: *Manual of structural kinesiology,* ed 12, St Louis, 1994, Mosby.)

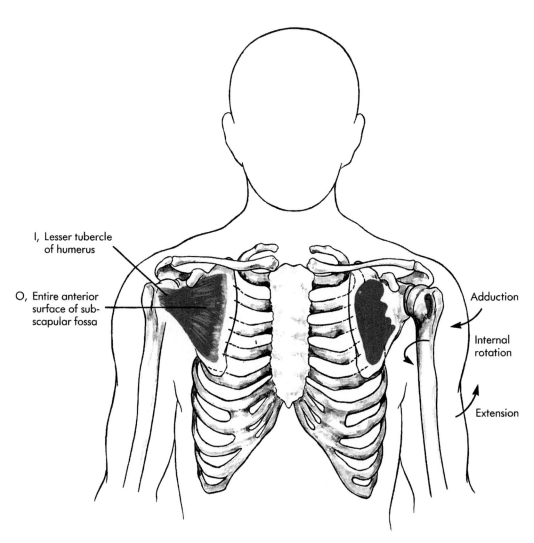

I, Lesser tubercle
of humerus

O, Entire anterior
surface of sub-
scapular fossa

Adduction

Internal
rotation

Extension

FIG 3-34. Subscapularis muscle. *O,* Origin; *I,* insertion. (From Thompson CW, Floyd RT: *Manual of structural kinesiology,* ed 12, St Louis, 1994, Mosby.)

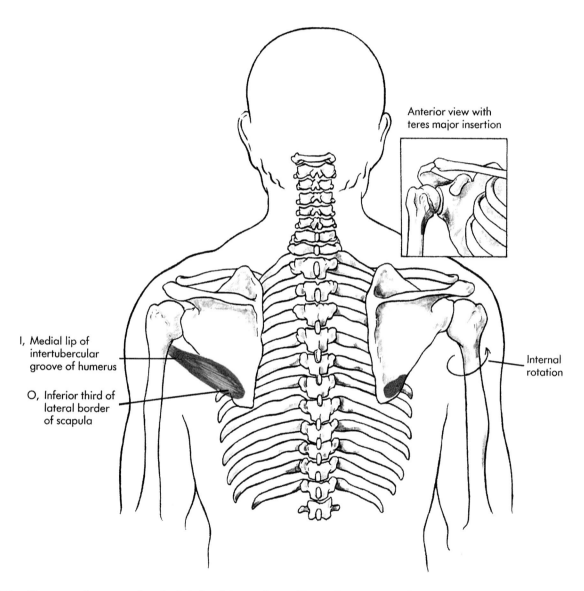

Anterior view with
teres major insertion

I, Medial lip of
intertubercular
groove of humerus

O, Inferior third of
lateral border
of scapula

Internal
rotation

IG 3-35.   Teres major muscle. *O,* Origin; *I,* insertion. (From Thompson CW, Floyd RT: *Manual of structural kinesiology,* ed 12, St Louis, 1994, Mosby.)

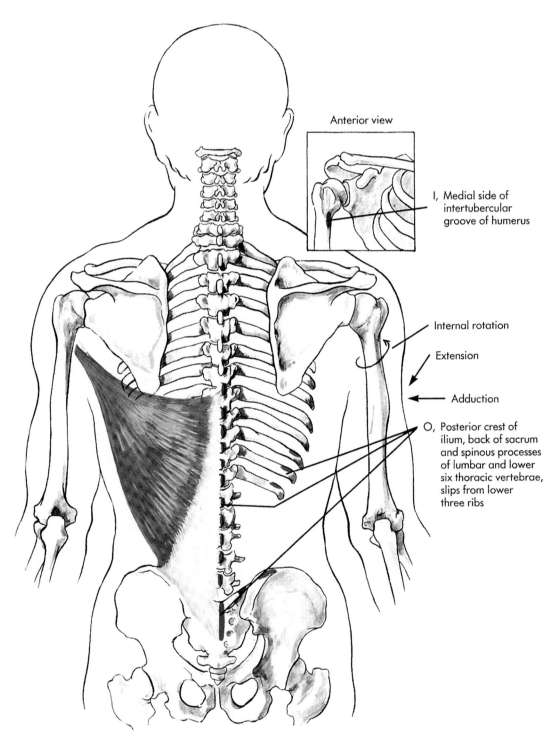

Anterior view

I, Medial side of
intertubercular
groove of humerus

Internal rotation

Extension

Adduction

O, Posterior crest of
ilium, back of sacrum
and spinous processes
of lumbar and lower
six thoracic vertebrae,
slips from lower
three ribs

FIG 3-36.   Latissimus dorsi muscle. *O,* Origin; *I,* insertion. (From Thompson CW, Floyd RT: *Manual of structural kinesiology,* ed 12, St Louis, 1994, Mosby.)

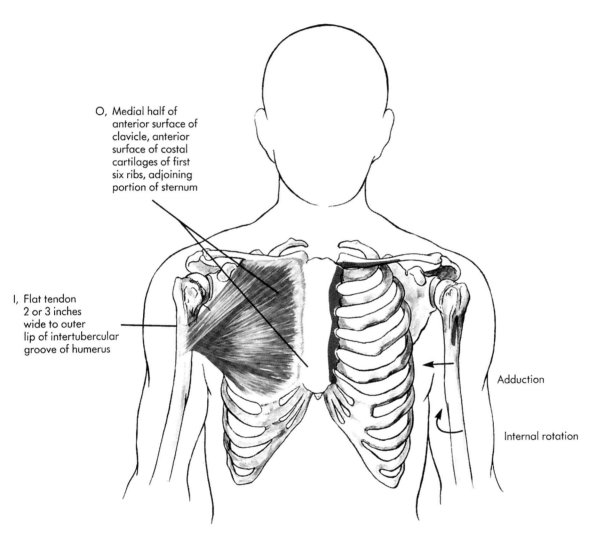

O, Medial half of anterior surface of clavicle, anterior surface of costal cartilages of first six ribs, adjoining portion of sternum

I, Flat tendon 2 or 3 inches wide to outer lip of intertubercular groove of humerus

Adduction

Internal rotation

FIG 3-37.   Pectoralis major muscle. *O,* Origin; *I,* insertion. (From Thompson CW, Floyd RT: *Manual of structural kinesiology,* ed 12, St Louis, 1994, Mosby.)

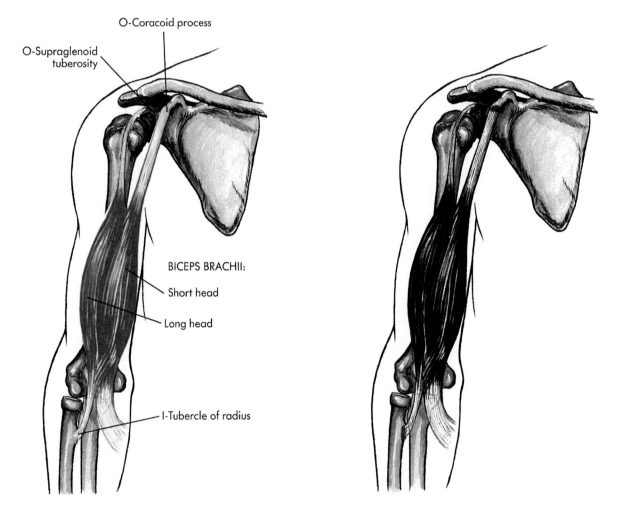

O-Coracoid process

O-Supraglenoid
tuberosity

BICEPS BRACHII:

Short head

Long head

I-Tubercle of radius

FIG 3-38.   Biceps brachii muscle. *O,* Origin; *I,* insertion. (From Thompson CW, Floyd RT: *Manual of structural kinesiology,* ed 12, St Louis, 1994, Mosby.)

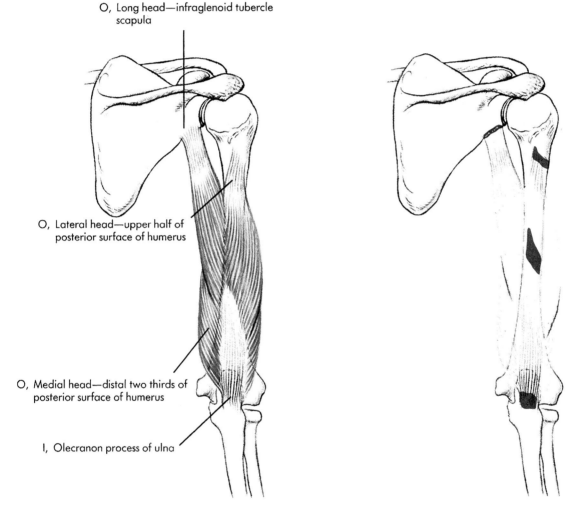

O, Long head—infraglenoid tubercle
   scapula

O, Lateral head—upper half of
   posterior surface of humerus

O, Medial head—distal two thirds of
   posterior surface of humerus

I, Olecranon process of ulna

FIG 3-39. Triceps brachii muscle. *O,* Origin; *I,* insertion. (From Thompson CW, Floyd RT: *Manual of structural kinesiology,* ed 12, St Louis, 1994, Mosby.)

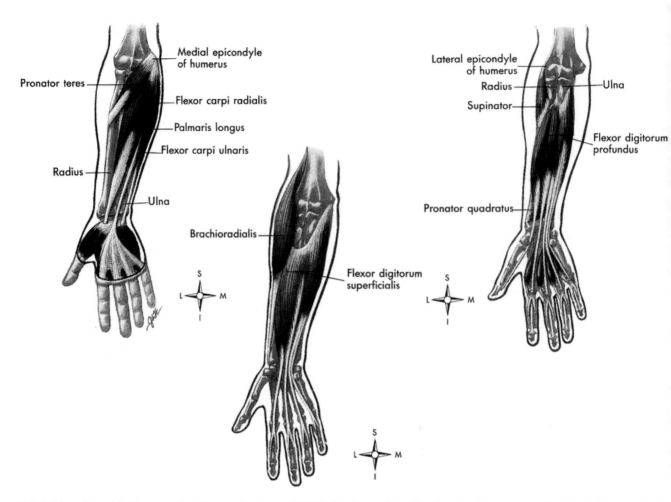

FIG 3-40.   Brachialis muscle. (From Anthony CP, Thibodeau GA: *Textbook of anatomy & physiology,* ed 12, St Louis, 1987, Mosby.)

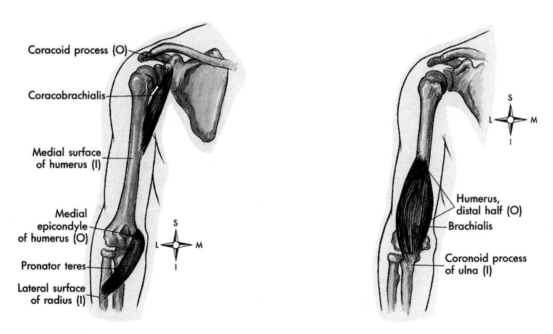

FIG 3-41.   Coracobrachialis and pronator teres muscles. (From Anthony CP, Thibodeau GA: *Textbook of anatomy & physiology,* ed 12, St Louis, 1987, Mosby.)

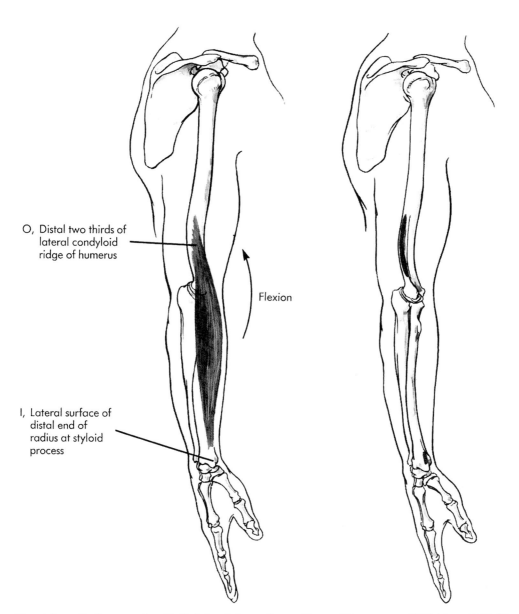

O, Distal two thirds of
lateral condyloid
ridge of humerus

Flexion

I, Lateral surface of
distal end of
radius at styloid
process

FIG 3-42.   Brachioradialis muscle. *O,* Origin; *I,* insertion. (From Thompson CW, Floyd RT: *Manual of structural kinesiology,* ed 12, St Louis, 1994, Mosby.)

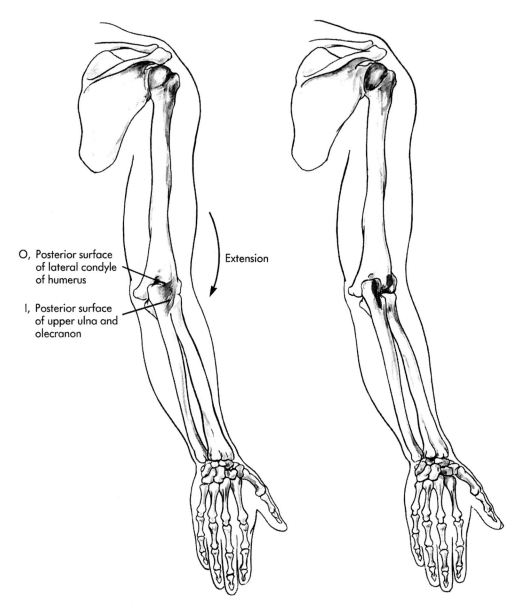

O, Posterior surface
of lateral condyle
of humerus

I, Posterior surface
of upper ulna and
olecranon

Extension

FIG 3-43. Anconeus muscle. *O,* Origin; *I,* insertion. (From Thompson CW, Floyd RT: *Manual of structural kinesiology,* ed 12, St Louis, 1994, Mosby.)

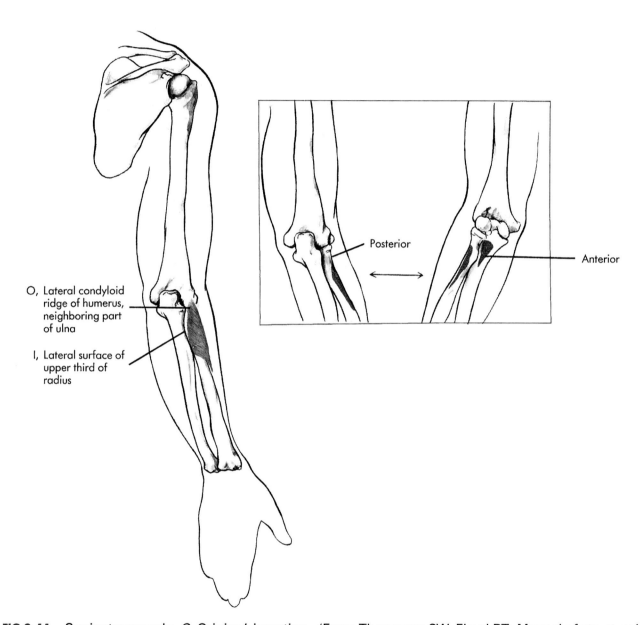

O, Lateral condyloid
ridge of humerus,
neighboring part
of ulna

I, Lateral surface of
upper third of
radius

Posterior

Anterior

FIG 3-44. Supinator muscle. *O,* Origin; *I,* insertion. (From Thompson CW, Floyd RT: *Manual of structural kinesiology,* ed 12, St Louis, 1994, Mosby.)

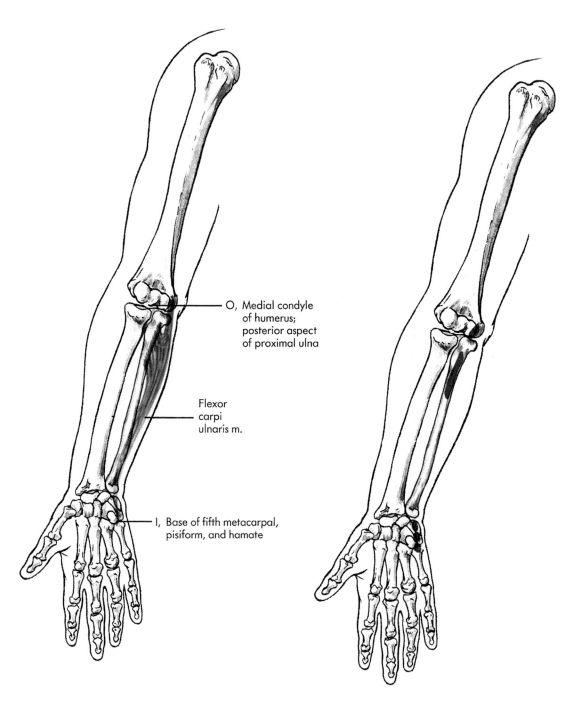

O, Medial condyle
of humerus;
posterior aspect
of proximal ulna

Flexor
carpi
ulnaris m.

I, Base of fifth metacarpal,
pisiform, and hamate

FIG 3-45.   Flexor carpi ulnaris muscle. *O,* Origin; *I,* insertion. (From Thompson CW, Floyd RT: *Manual of structural kinesiology,* ed 12, St Louis, 1994, Mosby.)

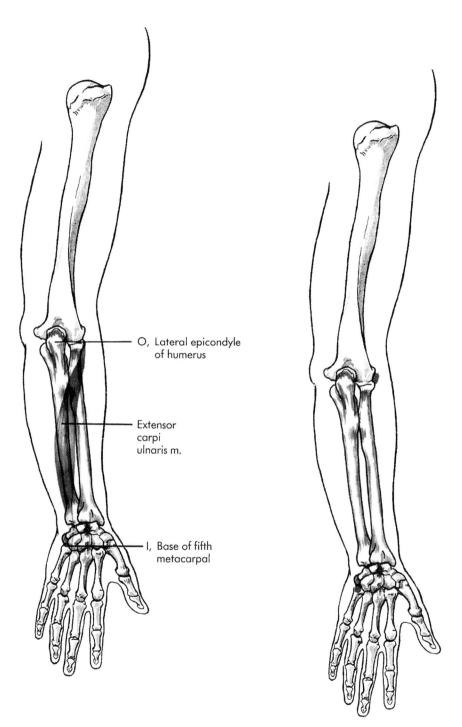

O, Lateral epicondyle of humerus

Extensor carpi ulnaris m.

I, Base of fifth metacarpal

FIG 3-46. Extensor carpi ulnaris muscle. *O,* Origin; *I,* insertion. (From Thompson CW, Floyd RT: *Manual of structural kinesiology,* ed 12, St Louis, 1994, Mosby.)

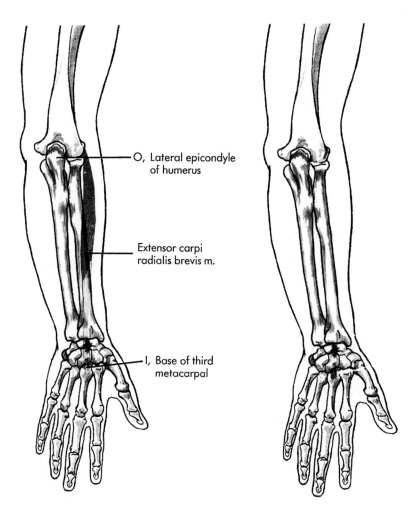

FIG 3-47. Extensor carpi radialis brevis muscle. *O,* Origin; *I,* insertion. (From Thompson CW, Floyd RT: *Manual of structural kinesiology,* ed 12, St Louis, 1994, Mosby.)

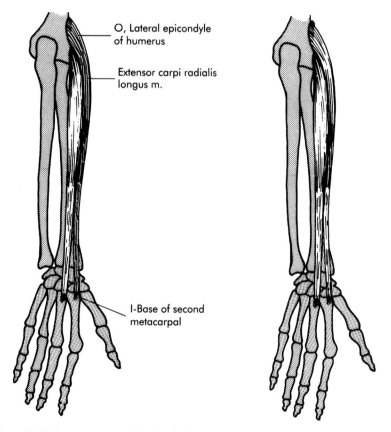

O, Lateral epicondyle
of humerus

Extensor carpi radialis
longus m.

I-Base of second
metacarpal

FIG 3-48.   Extensor carpi radialis longus muscle. *O,* Origin; *I,* insertion. (From Thompson CW, Floyd RT:
Manual of structural kinesiology, ed 12, St Louis, 1994, Mosby.)

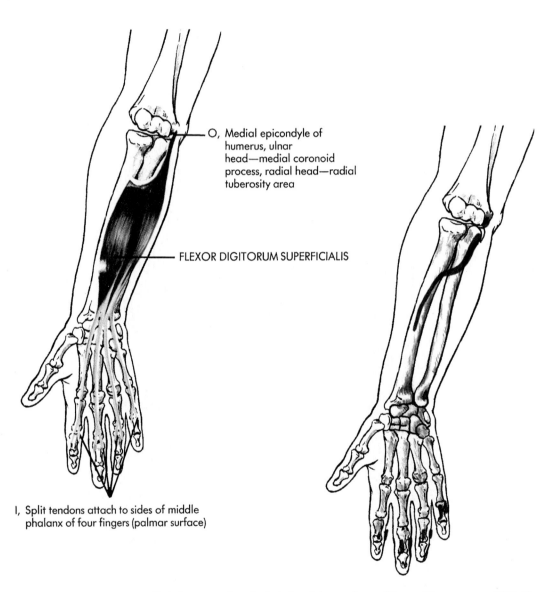

O, Medial epicondyle of
humerus, ulnar
head—medial coronoid
process, radial head—radial
tuberosity area

FLEXOR DIGITORUM SUPERFICIALIS

I, Split tendons attach to sides of middle
phalanx of four fingers (palmar surface)

FIG 3-49. Flexor digitorum superficialis muscle. *O,* Origin; *I,* insertion. (From Thompson CW, Floyd RT: *Manual of structural kinesiology,* ed 12, St Louis, 1994, Mosby.)

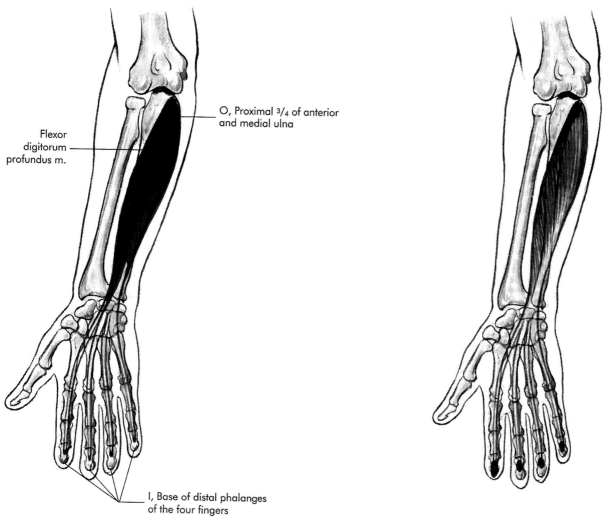

Flexor
digitorum
profundus m.

O, Proximal 3/4 of anterior
and medial ulna

I, Base of distal phalanges
of the four fingers

FIG 3-50.   Flexor digitorum profundus muscle. *O,* Origin; *I,* insertion. (From Thompson CW, Floyd RT: *Manual of structural kinesiology,* ed 12, St Louis, 1994, Mosby.)

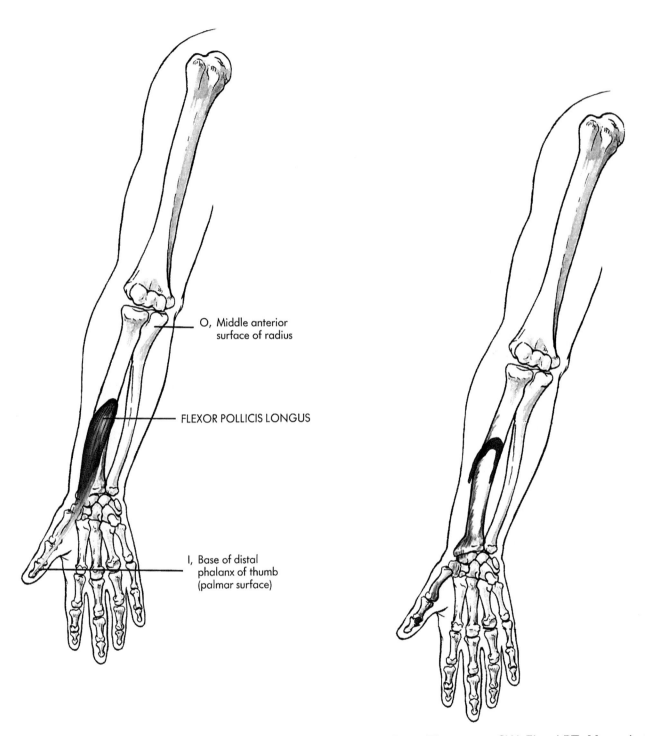

O, Middle anterior
surface of radius

FLEXOR POLLICIS LONGUS

I, Base of distal
phalanx of thumb
(palmar surface)

FIG 3-51. Flexor pollicis longus muscle. *O,* Origin; *I,* insertion. (From Thompson CW, Floyd RT: *Manual of structural kinesiology,* ed 12, St Louis, 1994, Mosby.)

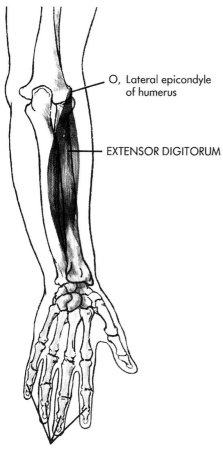

O, Lateral epicondyle
of humerus

EXTENSOR DIGITORUM

I, Four tendons to bases
of second and third phalanges
of four fingers (dorsal surface)

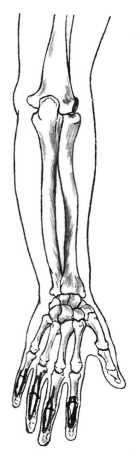

FIG 3-52. Extensor digitorum muscle. *O,* Origin; *I,* insertion. (From Thompson CW, Floyd RT: *Manual of structural kinesiology,* ed 12, St Louis, 1994, Mosby.)

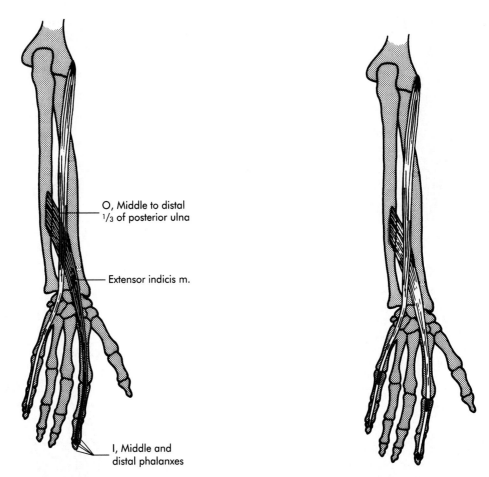

O, Middle to distal
⅓ of posterior ulna

Extensor indicis m.

I, Middle and
distal phalanxes

FIG 3-53. Extensor indicis muscle. *O,* Origin; *I,* insertion. (From Thompson CW, Floyd RT: *Manual of structural kinesiology,* ed 12, St Louis, 1994, Mosby.)

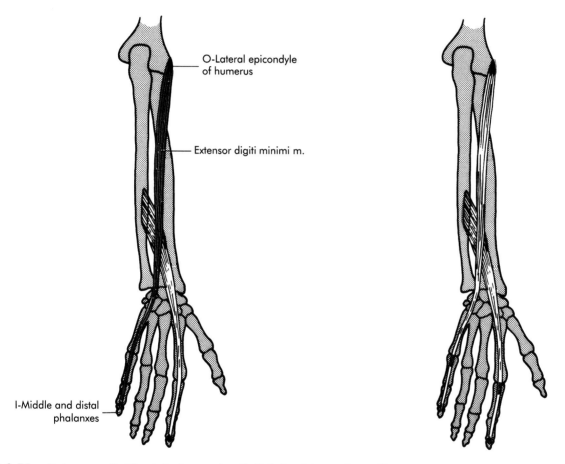

O-Lateral epicondyle
of humerus

Extensor digiti minimi m.

I-Middle and distal
phalanxes

FIG 3-54.   Extensor digiti minimi muscle. *O,* Origin; *I,* insertion. (From Thompson CW, Floyd RT: *Manual of structural kinesiology,* ed 12, St Louis, 1994, Mosby.)

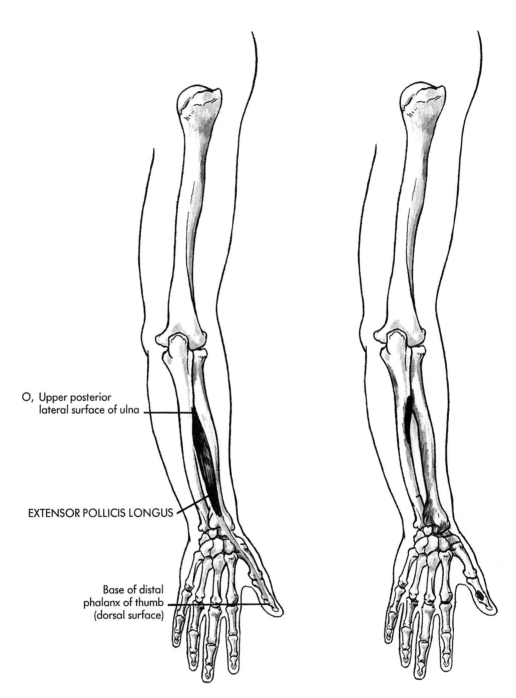

O, Upper posterior
lateral surface of ulna

EXTENSOR POLLICIS LONGUS

Base of distal
phalanx of thumb
(dorsal surface)

FIG 3-55.   Extensor pollicis longus muscle. *O,* Origin; *I,* insertion. (From Thompson CW, Floyd RT: *Manual of structural kinesiology,* ed 12, St Louis, 1994, Mosby.)

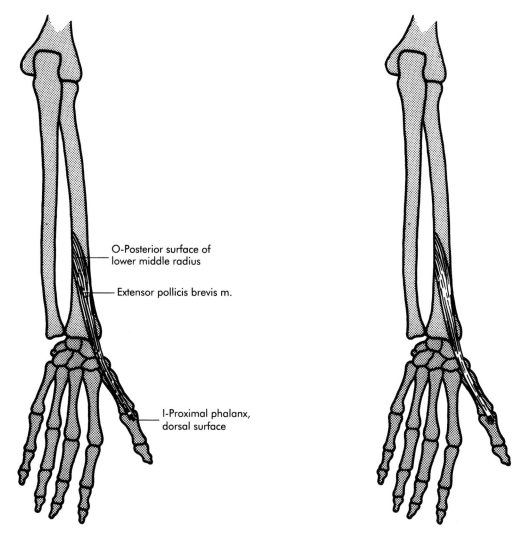

FIG 3-56. Extensor pollicis brevis muscle. *O,* Origin; *I,* insertion. (From Thompson CW, Floyd RT: *Manual of structural kinesiology,* ed 12, St Louis, 1994, Mosby.)

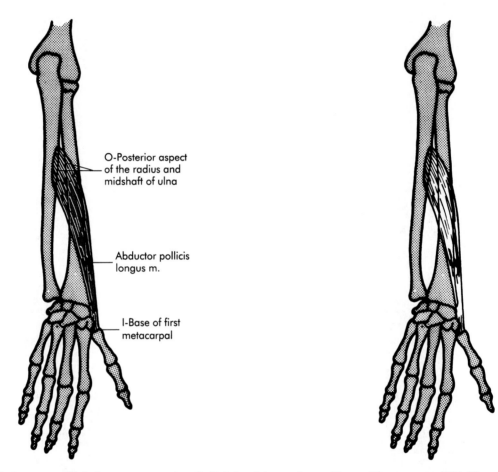

O-Posterior aspect
of the radius and
midshaft of ulna

Abductor pollicis
longus m.

I-Base of first
metacarpal

FIG 3-57.   Abductor pollicis longus muscle. *O,* Origin; *I,* insertion. (From Thompson CW, Floyd RT: *Manual of structural kinesiology,* ed 12, St Louis, 1994, Mosby.

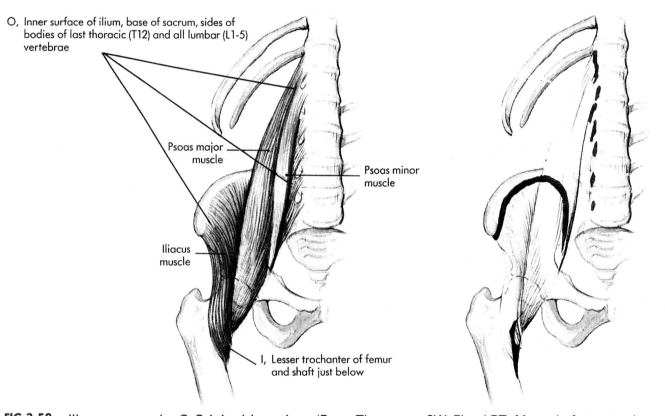

O, Inner surface of ilium, base of sacrum, sides of bodies of last thoracic (T12) and all lumbar (L1-5) vertebrae

Psoas major muscle

Psoas minor muscle

Iliacus muscle

I, Lesser trochanter of femur and shaft just below

FIG 3-58.   Iliopsoas muscle. *O,* Origin; *I,* insertion. (From Thompson CW, Floyd RT: *Manual of structural kinesiology,* ed 12, St Louis, 1994, Mosby.)

O, Notch between
anterior superior
and anterior inferior
spines of ilium

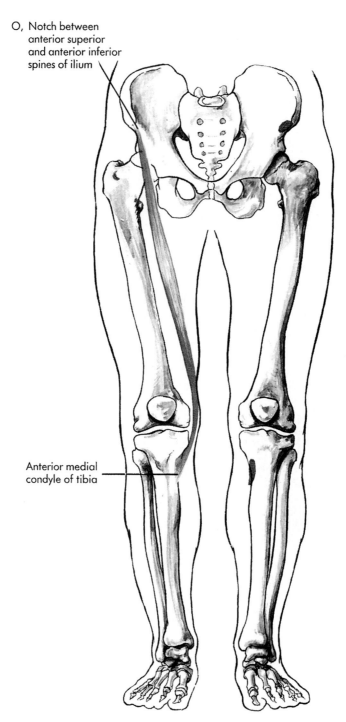

Anterior medial
condyle of tibia

FIG 3-59.   Sartorius muscle. *O,* Origin; *I,* insertion.   (From Thompson CW, Floyd RT: *Manual of structural kinesiology,* ed 12, St Louis, 1994, Mosby.)

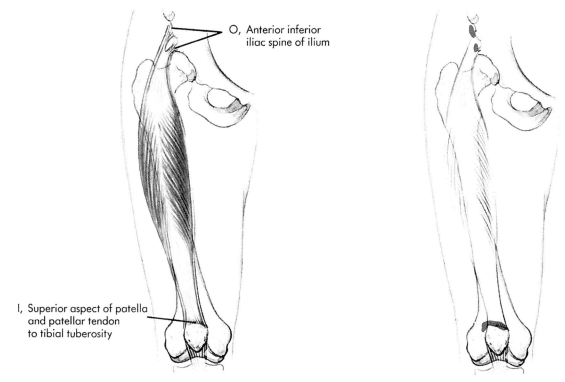

O, Anterior inferior
iliac spine of ilium

I, Superior aspect of patella
and patellar tendon
to tibial tuberosity

FIG 3-60.   Rectus femoris muscle. *O,* Origin; *I,* insertion. (From Thompson CW, Floyd RT: *Manual of structural kinesiology,* ed 12, St Louis, 1994, Mosby.)

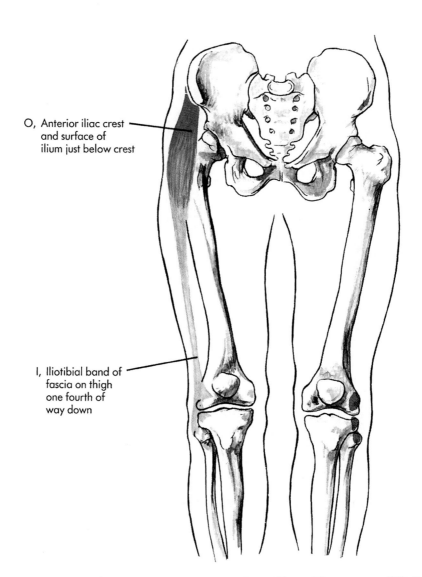

O, Anterior iliac crest
and surface of
ilium just below crest

I, Iliotibial band of
fascia on thigh
one fourth of
way down

FIG 3-61. Tensor fasciae latae muscle. *O,* Origin; *I,* insertion. (From Thompson CW, Floyd RT: *Manual of structural kinesiology,* ed 12, St Louis, 1994, Mosby.)

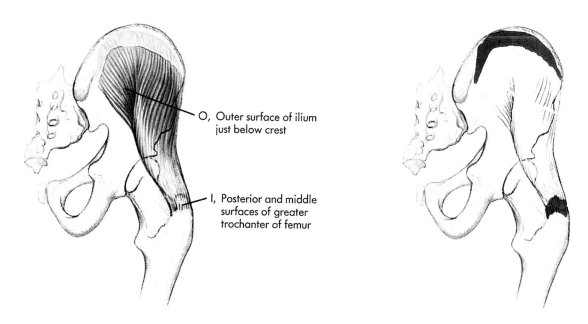

O, Outer surface of ilium
just below crest

I, Posterior and middle
surfaces of greater
trochanter of femur

FIG 3-62. Gluteus medius muscle. *O,* Origin; *I,* insertion. (From Thompson CW, Floyd RT: *Manual of structural kinesiology,* ed 12, St Louis, 1994, Mosby.)

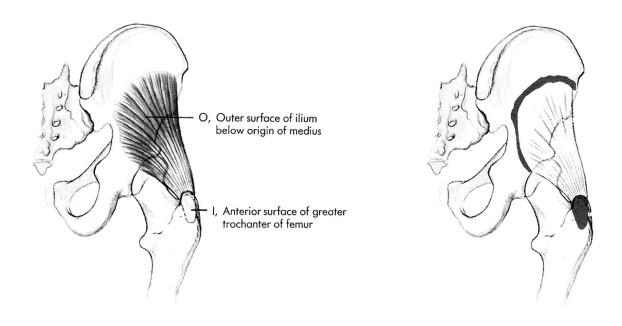

O, Outer surface of ilium
below origin of medius

I, Anterior surface of greater
trochanter of femur

FIG 3-63. Gluteus minimus muscle. *O,* Origin; *I,* insertion. (From Thompson CW, Floyd RT: *Manual of structural kinesiology,* ed 12, St Louis, 1994, Mosby.)

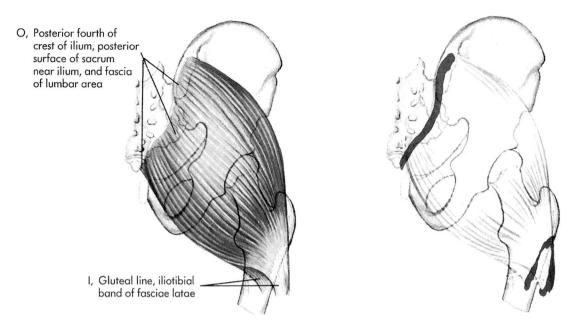

O, Posterior fourth of crest of ilium, posterior surface of sacrum near ilium, and fascia of lumbar area

I, Gluteal line, iliotibial band of fasciae latae

FIG 3-64. Gluteus maximus muscle. *O,* Origin; *I,* insertion. (From Thompson CW, Floyd RT: *Manual of structural kinesiology,* ed 12, St Louis, 1994, Mosby.)

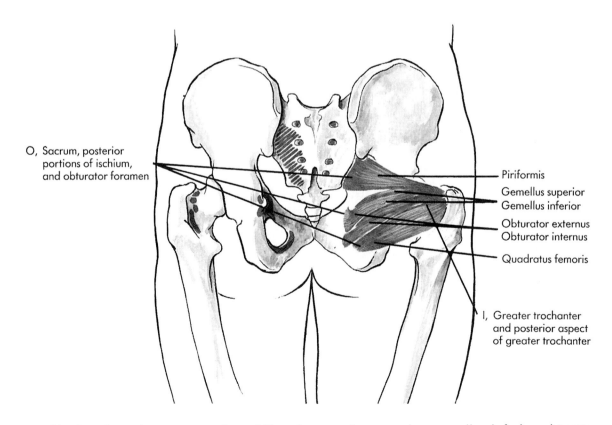

O, Sacrum, posterior portions of ischium, and obturator foramen

Piriformis
Gemellus superior
Gemellus inferior
Obturator externus
Obturator internus
Quadratus femoris

I, Greater trochanter and posterior aspect of greater trochanter

FIG 3-65. Six deep lateral rotator muscles: piriformis, gemellus superior, gemellus inferior, obturator externus, obturator internus, and quadratus femoris. (From Thompson CW, Floyd RT: *Manual of structural kinesiology,* ed 12, St Louis, 1994, Mosby.)

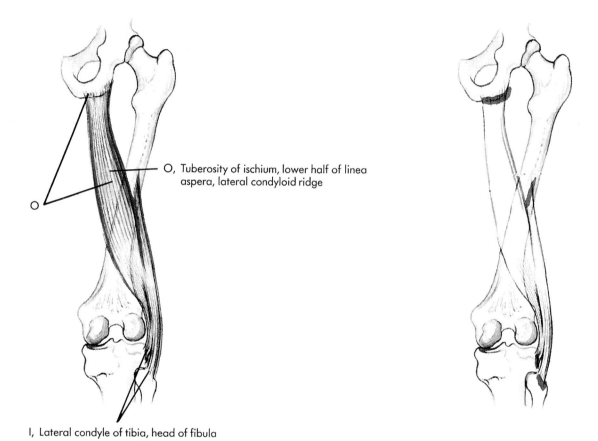

O, Tuberosity of ischium, lower half of linea aspera, lateral condyloid ridge

I, Lateral condyle of tibia, head of fibula

FIG 3-66. Biceps femoris muscle. *O,* Origin; *I,* insertion. (From Thompson CW, Floyd RT: *Manual of structural kinesiology,* ed 12, St Louis, 1994, Mosby.)

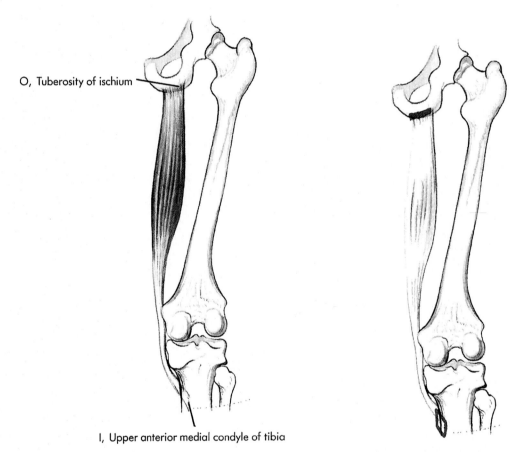

O, Tuberosity of ischium

I, Upper anterior medial condyle of tibia

FIG 3-67.   Semitendinosus muscle. *O,* Origin; *I,* insertion. (From Thompson CW, Floyd RT: *Manual of structural kinesiology,* ed 12, St Louis, 1994, Mosby.)

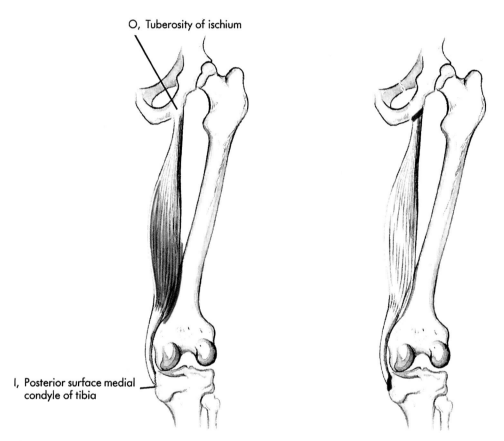

O, Tuberosity of ischium

I, Posterior surface medial condyle of tibia

FIG 3-68. Semimembranosus muscle. *O,* Origin; *I,* insertion. (From Thompson CW, Floyd RT: *Manual of structural kinesiology,* ed 12, St Louis, 1994, Mosby.)

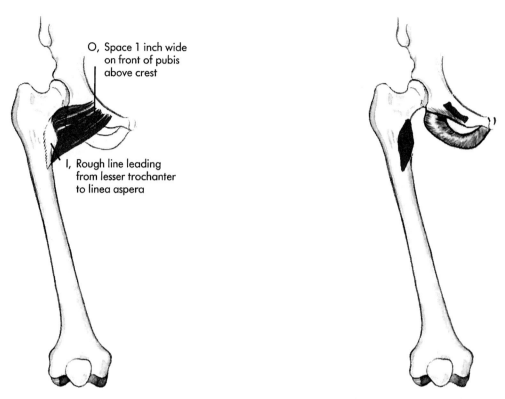

FIG 3-69. Pectineus muscle. *O,* Origin; *I,* insertion. (From Thompson CW, Floyd RT: *Manual of structural kinesiology,* ed 12, St Louis, 1994, Mosby.)

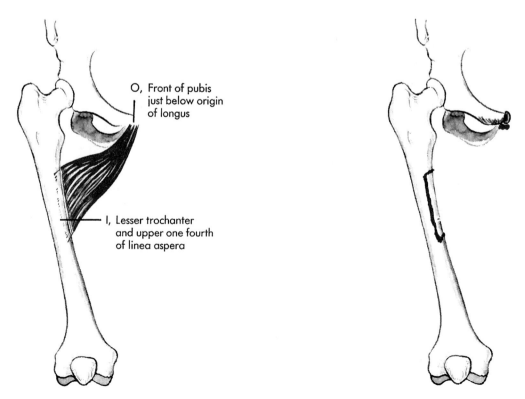

FIG 3-70. Adductor brevis muscle. *O,* Origin; *I,* insertion. (From Thompson CW, Floyd RT: *Manual of structural kinesiology,* ed 12, St Louis, 1994, Mosby.)

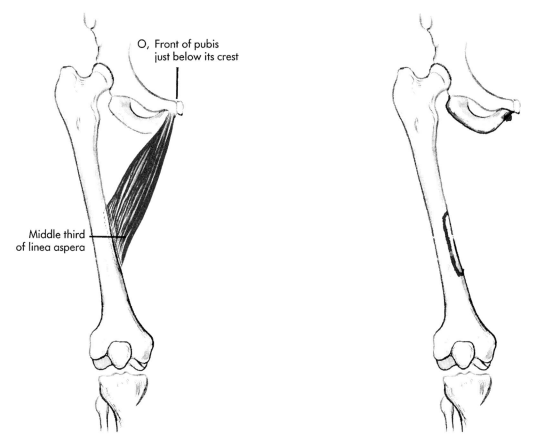

FIG 3-71. Adductor longus muscle. *O,* Origin; *I,* insertion. (From Thompson CW, Floyd RT: *Manual of structural kinesiology,* ed 12, St Louis, 1994, Mosby.)

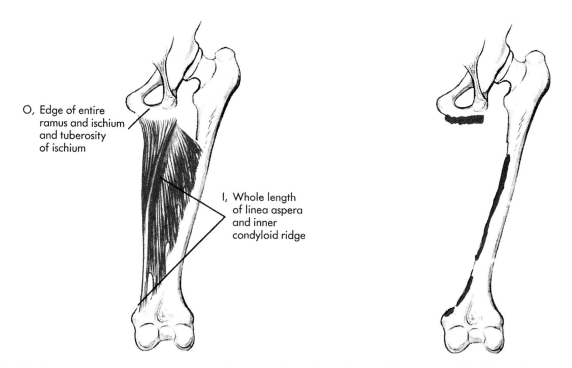

FIG 3-72. Adductor magnus muscle. *O,* Origin; *I,* insertion. (From Thompson CW, Floyd RT: *Manual of structural kinesiology,* ed 12, St Louis, 1994, Mosby.)

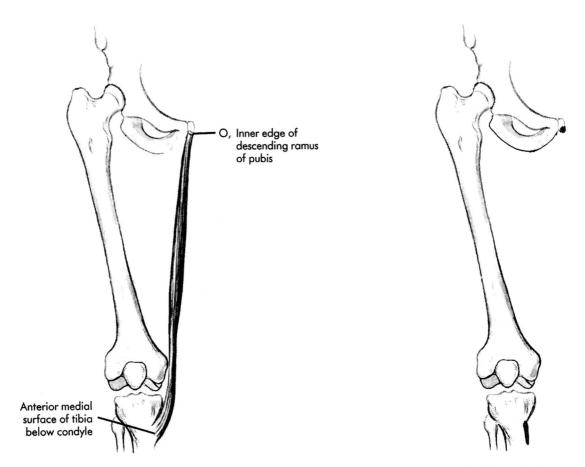

O, Inner edge of
descending ramus
of pubis

Anterior medial
surface of tibia
below condyle

FIG 3-73. Gracilis muscle. *O,* Origin; *I,* insertion. (From Thompson CW, Floyd RT: *Manual of structural kinesiology,* ed 12, St Louis, 1994, Mosby.)

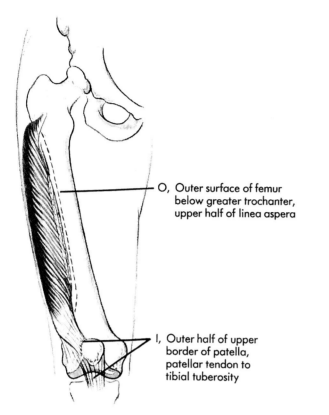
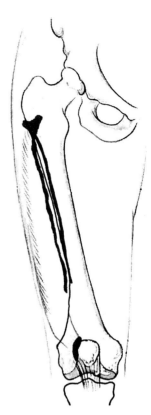

O, Outer surface of femur
below greater trochanter,
upper half of linea aspera

I, Outer half of upper
border of patella,
patellar tendon to
tibial tuberosity

FIG 3-74.   Vastus lateralis muscle. *O,* Origin; *I,* insertion. (From Thompson CW, Floyd RT: *Manual of structural kinesiology,* ed 12, St Louis, 1994, Mosby.)

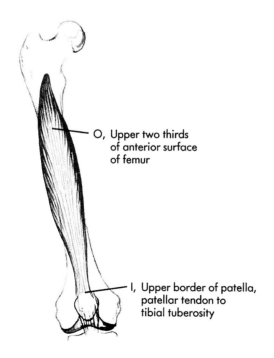
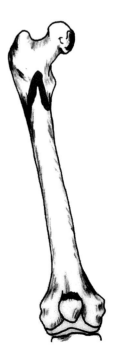

O, Upper two thirds
of anterior surface
of femur

I, Upper border of patella,
patellar tendon to
tibial tuberosity

FIG 3-75.   Vastus intermedius muscle. *O,* Origin; *I,* insertion. (From Thompson CW, Floyd RT: *Manual of structural kinesiology,* ed 12, St Louis, 1994, Mosby.)

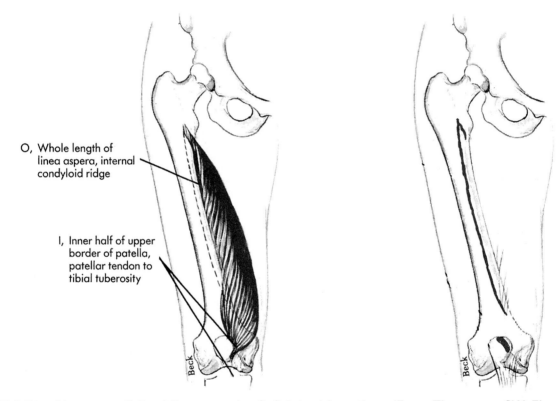

O, Whole length of linea aspera, internal condyloid ridge

I, Inner half of upper border of patella, patellar tendon to tibial tuberosity

Beck

FIG 3-76. Vastus medialis oblique muscle. *O,* Origin; *I,* insertion. (From Thompson CW, Floyd RT: *Manual of structural kinesiology,* ed 12, St Louis, 1994, Mosby.)

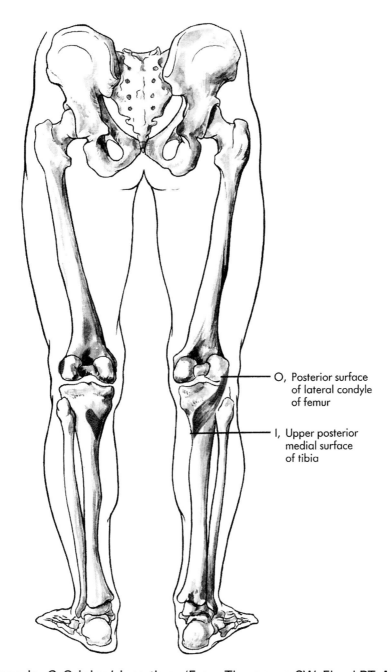

O, Posterior surface
of lateral condyle
of femur

I, Upper posterior
medial surface
of tibia

FIG 3-77. Popliteus muscle. *O,* Origin; *I,* insertion. (From Thompson CW, Floyd RT: *Manual of structural kinesiology,* ed 12, St Louis, 1994, Mosby.)

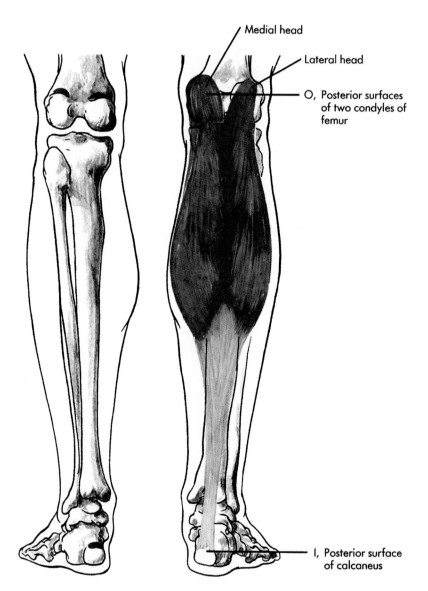

Medial head

Lateral head

O, Posterior surfaces
of two condyles of
femur

I, Posterior surface
of calcaneus

FIG 3-78.   Gastrocnemius muscle. *O,* Origin; *I,* insertion. (From Thompson CW, Floyd RT: *Manual of structural kinesiology,* ed 12, St Louis, 1994, Mosby.)

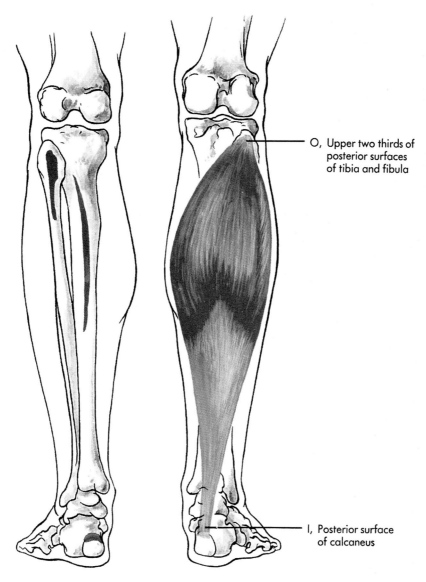

O, Upper two thirds of
posterior surfaces
of tibia and fibula

I, Posterior surface
of calcaneus

FIG 3-79.   Soleus muscle. *O,* Origin; *I,* insertion. (From Thompson CW, Floyd RT: *Manual of structural kinesiology,* ed 12, St Louis, 1994, Mosby.)

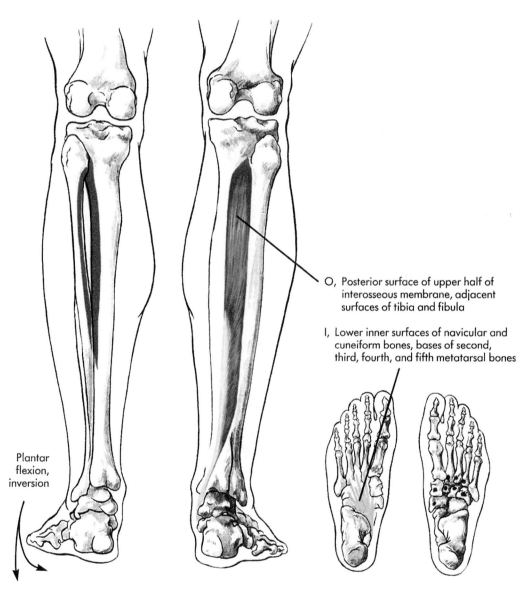

Plantar
flexion,
inversion

O, Posterior surface of upper half of
interosseous membrane, adjacent
surfaces of tibia and fibula

I, Lower inner surfaces of navicular and
cuneiform bones, bases of second,
third, fourth, and fifth metatarsal bones

FIG 3-80.   Tibialis posterior muscle. *O,* Origin; *I,* insertion. (From Thompson CW, Floyd RT: *Manual of structural kinesiology,* ed 12, St Louis, 1994, Mosby.)

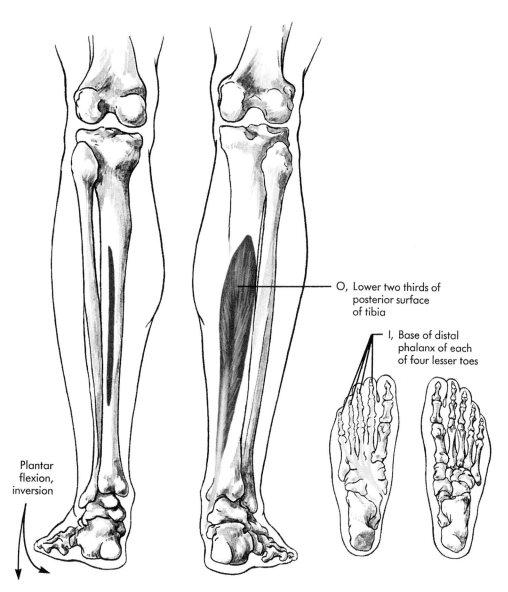

O, Lower two thirds of
posterior surface
of tibia

I, Base of distal
phalanx of each
of four lesser toes

Plantar
flexion,
inversion

FIG 3-81.   Flexor digitorum longus muscle. *O,* Origin; *I,* insertion. (From Thompson CW, Floyd RT: *Manual of structural kinesiology,* ed 12, St Louis, 1994, Mosby.)

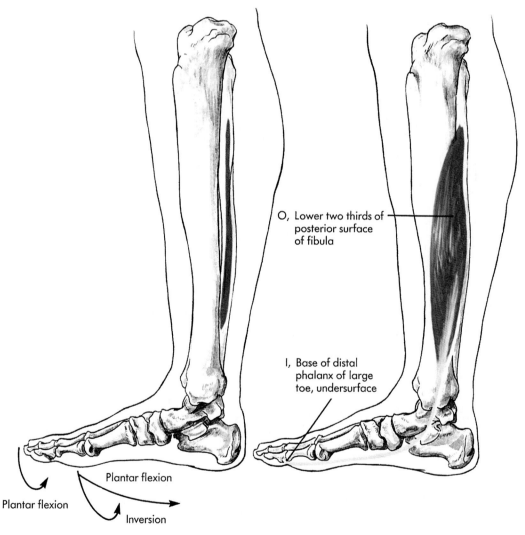

O, Lower two thirds of posterior surface of fibula

I, Base of distal phalanx of large toe, undersurface

Plantar flexion

Plantar flexion

Inversion

FIG 3-82. Flexor hallucis longus muscle. *O,* Origin; *I,* insertion. (From Thompson CW, Floyd RT: *Manual of structural kinesiology,* ed 12, St Louis, 1994, Mosby.)

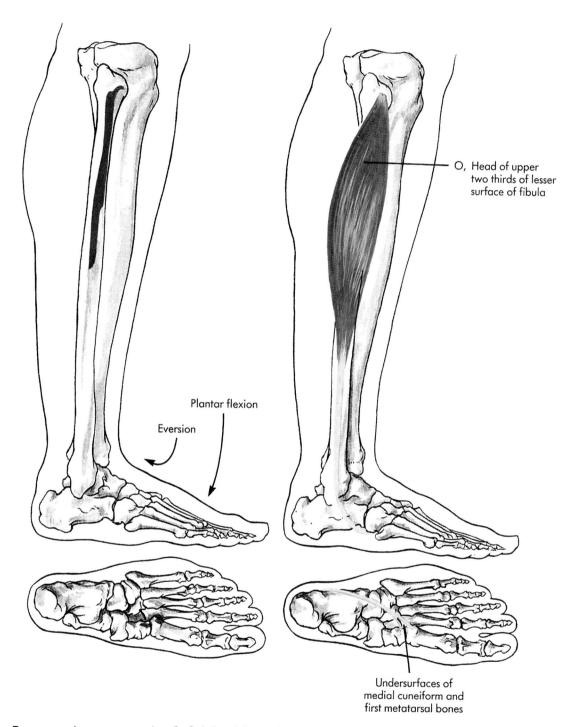

O, Head of upper
two thirds of lesser
surface of fibula

Plantar flexion

Eversion

Undersurfaces of
medial cuneiform and
first metatarsal bones

FIG 3-83.   Peroneus longus muscle. *O,* Origin; *I,* insertion. (From Thompson CW, Floyd RT: *Manual of structural kinesiology,* ed 12, St Louis, 1994, Mosby.)

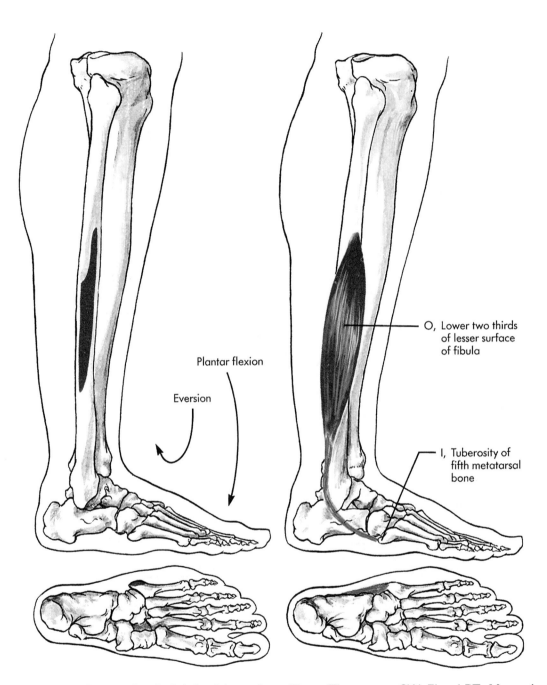

Plantar flexion

Eversion

O, Lower two thirds
of lesser surface
of fibula

I, Tuberosity of
fifth metatarsal
bone

FIG 3-84.   Peroneus brevis muscle. *O,* Origin; *I,* insertion. (From Thompson CW, Floyd RT: *Manual of structural kinesiology,* ed 12, St Louis, 1994, Mosby.)

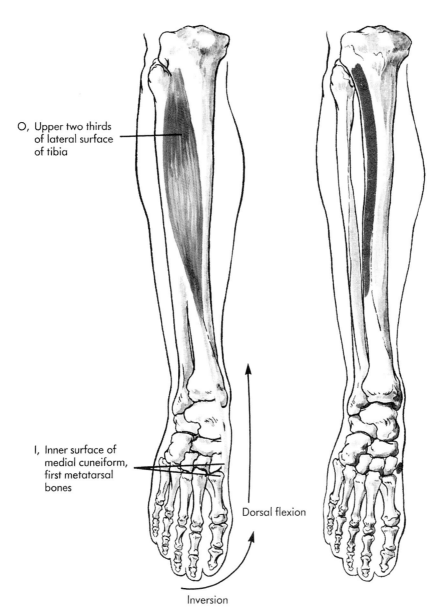

O, Upper two thirds
of lateral surface
of tibia

I, Inner surface of
medial cuneiform,
first metatarsal
bones

Dorsal flexion

Inversion

FIG 3-85. Tibialis anterior muscle. *O,* Origin; *I,* insertion. (From Thompson CW, Floyd RT: *Manual of structural kinesiology,* ed 12, St Louis, 1994, Mosby.)

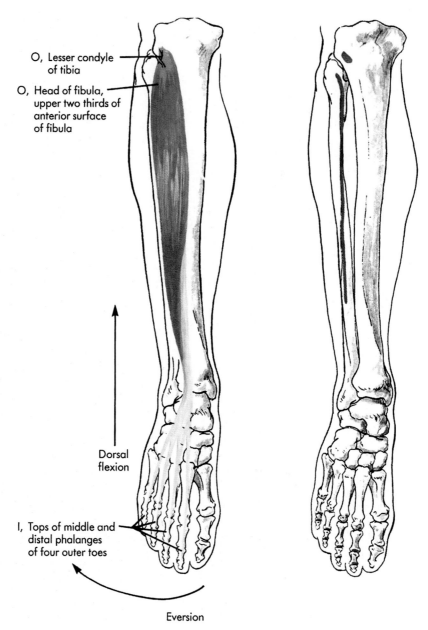

O, Lesser condyle
   of tibia

O, Head of fibula,
   upper two thirds of
   anterior surface
   of fibula

Dorsal
flexion

I, Tops of middle and
   distal phalanges
   of four outer toes

Eversion

FIG 3-86.   Extensor digitorum longus muscle. *O,* Origin; *I,* insertion. (From Thompson CW, Floyd RT: *Manual of structural kinesiology,* ed 12, St Louis, 1994, Mosby.)

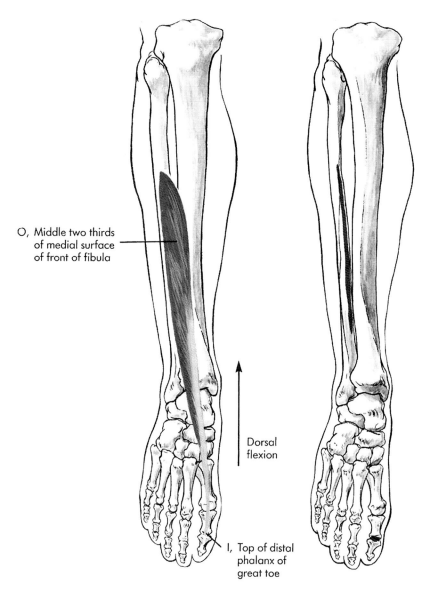

O, Middle two thirds
of medial surface
of front of fibula

Dorsal
flexion

I, Top of distal
phalanx of
great toe

FIG 3-87. Extensor hallucis longus muscle. *O,* Origin; *I,* insertion. (From Thompson CW, Floyd RT: *Manual of structural kinesiology,* ed 12, St Louis, 1994, Mosby.)

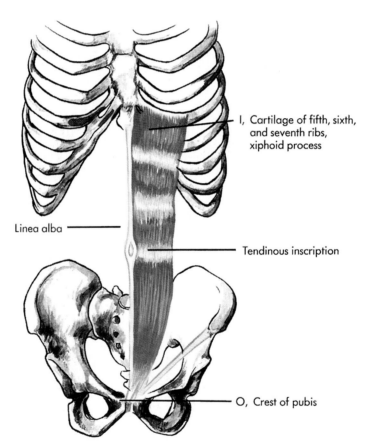

FIG 3-88. Rectus abdominis muscle. *O,* Origin; *I,* insertion. (From Thompson CW, Floyd RT: *Manual of structural kinesiology,* ed 12, St Louis, 1994, Mosby.)

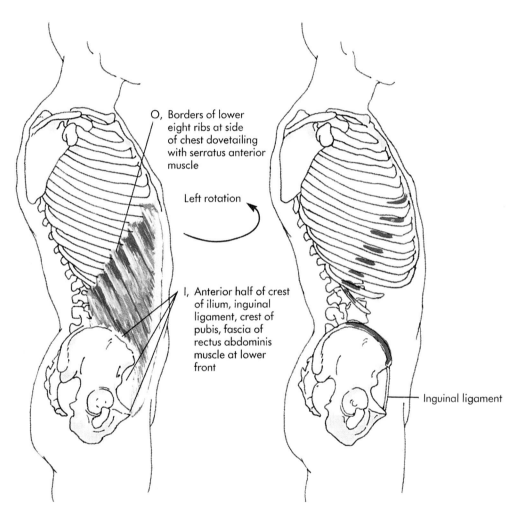

O, Borders of lower
eight ribs at side
of chest dovetailing
with serratus anterior
muscle

Left rotation

I, Anterior half of crest
of ilium, inguinal
ligament, crest of
pubis, fascia of
rectus abdominis
muscle at lower
front

Inguinal ligament

FIG 3-89.   External oblique muscle. *O,* Origin; *I,* insertion. (From Thompson CW, Floyd RT: *Manual of structural kinesiology,* ed 12, St Louis, 1994, Mosby.)

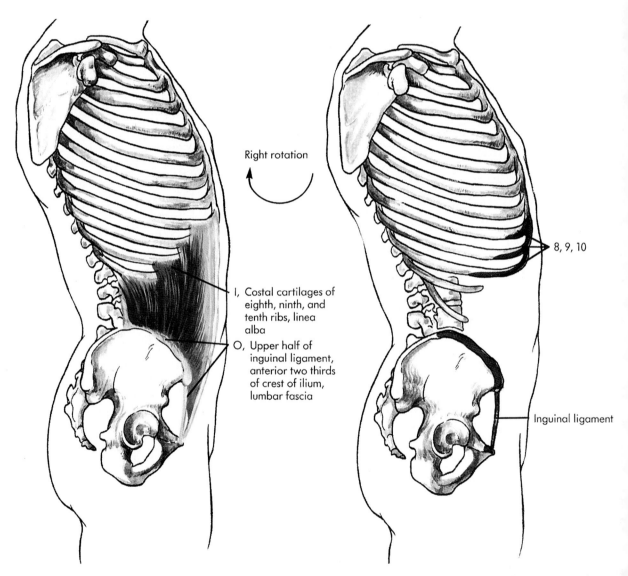

Right rotation

8, 9, 10

I, Costal cartilages of
eighth, ninth, and
tenth ribs, linea
alba

O, Upper half of
inguinal ligament,
anterior two thirds
of crest of ilium,
lumbar fascia

Inguinal ligament

FIG 3-90. Internal oblique muscle. *O,* Origin; *I,* insertion. (From Thompson CW, Floyd RT: *Manual of structural kinesiology,* ed 12, St Louis, 1994, Mosby.)

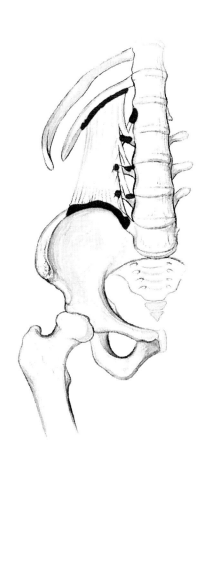

I, Transverse processes of upper four lumbar
vertebrae and lower border of twelfth rib

Quadratus
lumborum
muscle

O, Posterior inner lip of iliac crest

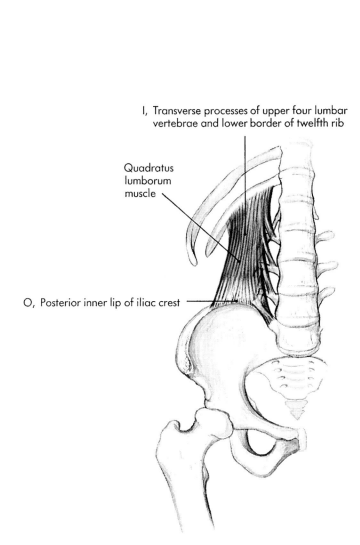

FIG 3-91.   Quadratus lumborum muscle. *O,* Origin; *I,* insertion. (From Thompson CW, Floyd RT: *Manual of structural kinesiology,* ed 12, St Louis, 1994, Mosby.)

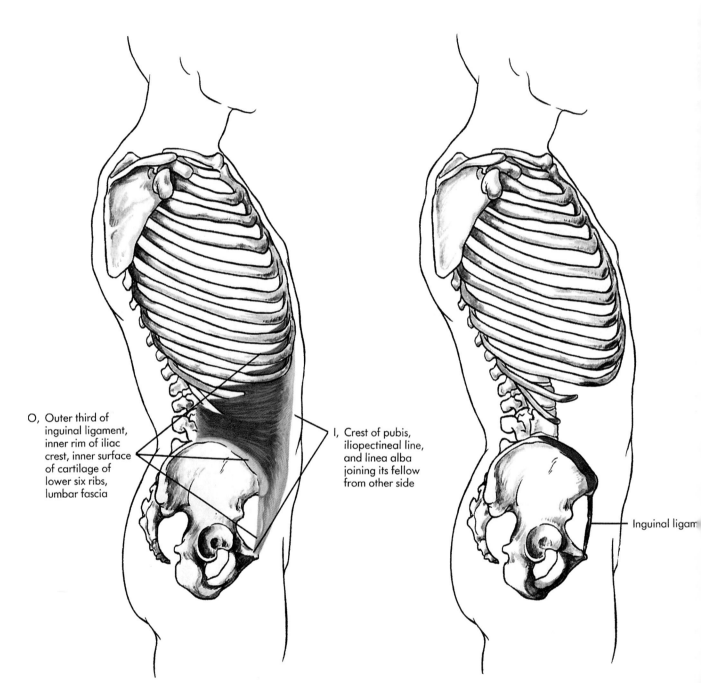

O, Outer third of inguinal ligament, inner rim of iliac crest, inner surface of cartilage of lower six ribs, lumbar fascia

I, Crest of pubis, iliopectineal line, and linea alba joining its fellow from other side

Inguinal ligam

FIG 3-92. Transversus abdominis muscle. *O,* Origin; *I,* insertion. (From Thompson CW, Floyd RT: *Manual of structural kinesiology,* ed 12, St Louis, 1994, Mosby.)

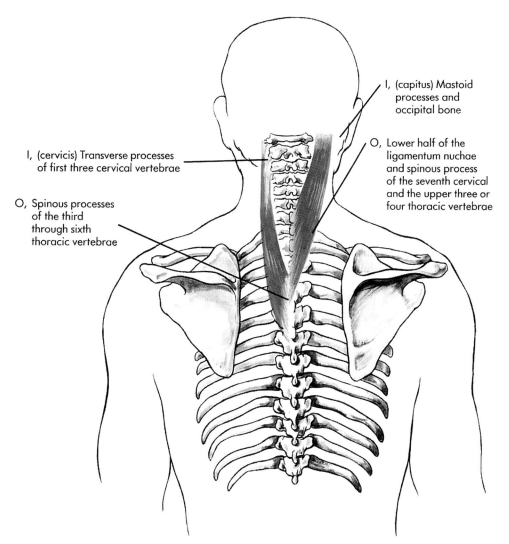

I, (capitus) Mastoid
processes and
occipital bone

O, Lower half of the
ligamentum nuchae
and spinous process
of the seventh cervical
and the upper three or
four thoracic vertebrae

I, (cervicis) Transverse processes
of first three cervical vertebrae

O, Spinous processes
of the third
through sixth
thoracic vertebrae

FIG 3-93.   Splenius muscles (splenius cervicis on the left, splenius capitis on the right). *O,* Origin; *I,*
insertion. (From Thompson CW, Floyd RT: *Manual of structural kinesiology,* ed 12, St Louis, 1994, Mosby.)

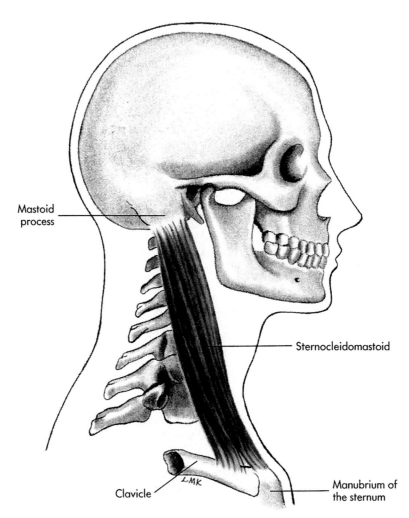

FIG 3-94. Sternocleidomastoid muscle. (From Thompson CW, Floyd RT: *Manual of structural kinesiology,* ed 12, St Louis, 1994, Mosby.)

Major Ligaments and Their Function

Joint	Ligament	Function
Shoulder girdle	Coracoclavicular	Holds clavicle to coracoid process
	Costoclavicular	Holds clavicle to costal cartilage of first rib
Shoulder joint	Coracohumeral	Strengthens upper portion of joint capsule
	Glenohumeral	Reinforces anterior aspect of joint capsule
	Coracoacromial	Protects superior aspect of joint
Elbow joint	Annular	Holds head of radius in position
	Ulnar collateral	Restricts medial displacement of elbow joint
	Radial collateral	Restricts lateral displacement of elbow joint
Wrist	Volar and dorsal radioulnar	Holds distal ends of radius and ulna in place
	Flexor and extensor retinacula	Holds tendons against bones
	Interosseous	Holds carpal bones together
	Dorsal and volar collateral	Connects articulations between rows of carpal bones
Fingers	Volar and collateral interphalangeal	Prevents displacement of interphalangeal joints
Ischium	Sacrospinous	Runs from sacrum to ischial spine to create greater sciatic foramen
	Sacrotuberous	Runs from sacrum to ischial tuberosity and prevents sacrum from tilting
Pubis	Transverse	Converts acetabular notch into foramen
	Superior pubic	Holds pubic bones together
	Arcuate pubic	Holds pubic bones together
Hip joint	Ligamentum teres	Carries nutrient vessels into head of femur
	Transverse	Holds femoral head in place
	Iliofemoral	Limits extension of hip
	Ischiofemoral	Limits anterior displacement of hip
	Pubofemoral	Limits extension of hip
Knee joint	Medial collateral	Stabilizes medial aspect of knee joint (tibiofemoral joint)
	Lateral collateral	Stabilizes lateral aspect of knee joint
	Medial and lateral menisci	Provides stability and cushions tibiofemoral articulation
	Anterior cruciate	Prevents backward sliding of femur and hyperextension of knee
	Posterior cruciate	Prevents forward sliding of femur
	Oblique and arcuate popliteal	Provides lateral and posterior support to knee joint
Ankle	Deltoid	Provides stability between medial malleolus, navicular bone, talus, and calcaneus
	Anterior and posterior talofibular	Secures fibula to talus
	Calcaneofibular	Secures fibula to calcaneus
Intertarsal	Long plantar	Provides groove for peroneus longus tendon and runs from calcaneus to metatarsals
	Calcaneonavicular	Supports head of talus between navicular bone and calcaneus
Tarsometatarsal	Dorsal and plantar interosseus	Limits movement of tarsal bones
Intermetatarsal	Dorsal and plantar transmetatarsal	Limits movement of metatarsal bones
Metatarsophalangeal	Plantar and transverse metatarsal	Holds metatarsophalangeal joints in place

NERVOUS SYSTEM

Muscles and Innervating Brachial Plexus Nerves

Nerve	Spinal cord segment(s)	Muscle(s)
Dorsal scapular	C4, C5	Rhomboid major
Long thoracic	C5, C6, C7	Serratus anterior
Suprascapular	C4, C5, C6	Supraspinatus
		Infraspinatus
Subscapular	C5, C6	Teres major
		Subscapularis
Anterior thoracic	C5 through T1	Pectoralis minor
		Pectoralis major
Musculocutaneous	C5, C6, C7	Biceps brachii
		Coracobrachialis
Radial	C5 through T1	Triceps brachii
		Brachialis
		Brachioradialis
		Supinator
		Extensor carpi radialis longus
		Extensor carpi radialis brevis
		Extensor carpi ulnaris
		Extensor digitorum
		Extensor pollicis longus
		Extensor pollicis brevis
		Extensor indicis
		Abductor pollicis longus
Median	C5 through T1	Pronator teres
		Pronator quadratus
		Palmaris longus
		Flexor carpi radialis
		Flexor digitorum
		Flexor digitorum profundus (radial half)
		Flexor pollicis longus
		Flexor pollicis brevis (shared with ulnar nerve)
		Abductor pollicis brevis
		Opponens pollicis
		Lumbrical muscles (on radial side of hand)
Ulnar	C7, C8, T1	Flexor carpi ulnaris
		Flexor digitorum profundus (ulnar half)
		Flexor pollicis brevis (shared with median nerve)
		Flexor digiti minimi brevis
		Abductor digiti minimi
		Adductor pollicis
		Opponens digiti minimi
		Lumbrical muscles (on ulnar side of hand)
		Interossei

Muscles and Innervating Nerves of the Lumbar and Sacral Plexuses

Nerve	Spinal cord segment(s)	Muscle(s)
Lumbar plexus		
Obturator	L2, L3, L4	Pectineus (shared with femoral nerve)
		Adductor longus
		Adductor magnus (shared with sciatic nerve)
		Adductor brevis
		Gracilis
Femoral	L2, L3, L4	Sartorius
		Iliacus
		Pectineus (shared with obturator nerve)
		Quadriceps femoris
		Rectus femoris
		Vastus medialis
		Vastus lateralis
		Vastus intermedius
Other muscular branches	L2, L3, L4	Psoas major
		Quadratus lumborum
Sacral plexus		
Superior gluteal	L4, L5, S1	Gluteus medius
		Gluteus minimus
		Tensor fasciae latae
Inferior gluteal	L5, S1, S2	Gluteus maximus
Sciatic	L4 through S3	Adductor magnus (shared with obturator nerve)
		Obturator internus
		Superior gemellus
		Inferior gemellus
		Quadratus femoris
Tibial portion of sciatic	L4 through S3	Biceps femoris (shared with peroneal nerve)
		Semitendinosus
		Semimembranosus
		Gastrocnemius
		Soleus
		Popliteus
		Tibialis posterior
		Flexor digitorum longus
		Flexor hallucis longus
		Plantar and medial foot muscles
Pudendal	S2, S3, S4	Muscles of urogenital triangle
Other muscular branches	S3, S4	Levator ani
		Coccygeus
		External anal sphincter

Innervation Levels of Various Muscle Groups

Muscle group	Innervation level
Trapezius	C3-5
Deltoids	C5-6
Biceps	C5-6
Internal rotators	C5-T1
External rotators	C5-6
Pectoralis major	C5-T1
Latissimus dorsi	C7-8

Muscle group	Innervation level
Triceps	C7-8
Supinators	C5-6
Pronators	C6-7
Extensor carpi radialis longus	C6-7
Extensor carpi ulnaris	C7-8
Flexor carpi radialis	C7-8
Flexor carpi ulnaris	C8
Flexor digitorum superficialis	C8-T1
Lumbricales	C8-T1
Interossei	C8-T1
Rectus abdominis	T7-12
Internal oblique	T7-L1
External oblique	T5-11
Sartorius	L1-3
Adductors	L2-4
External rotators	L3-S2
Internal rotators	L4-S1
Tensor fasciae latae	L4-S1
Hamstrings	L4-S3
Quadriceps	L2-4
Anterior tibialis	L4-5
Gastrocnemius	L5-S1
Flexor hallucis longus	S1-2
Extensor digitorum brevis	S2-3

Sensory Innervation Levels

Innervation level	Anatomical region
C1	Top of head
C2	Temple, forehead, occiput
C3	Neck, posterior cheek
C4	Superior part of chest above the axilla (clavicle area)
C5	Deltoid area of lateral arm
C6	Anterior arm, radial (lateral) side of hand to thumb and index finger
C7	Lateral arm and forearm to index, long, and ring fingers
C8	Middle arm and forearm to long, ring, and little fingers
T1	Medial side of forearm to base of little finger
T2	Chest at axilla level
T4	Level of nipple line
T6	Level of xiphoid process
T10	Level of umbilicus
T12	Level of anterior superior iliac crests
L1	Lower abdomen and groin (over trochanter)
L2	Anterolateral thigh (back and front of thigh to knee)
L3	Anteromedial thigh, leg, upper buttock
L4	Medial buttock, lateral thigh, medial leg, dorsum of foot, large toe
L5	Posterior, lateral thigh; lateral leg; dorsum of foot; medial half of sole; first, second, and third toes
S1	Lateral-plantar surface of foot, posterior thigh and leg
S2	Posterior thigh and leg
S3	Groin, medial thigh to knee
S4-5	Perineum, genitals, lower sacrum

Dermatomal Map (Fig. 3-95)

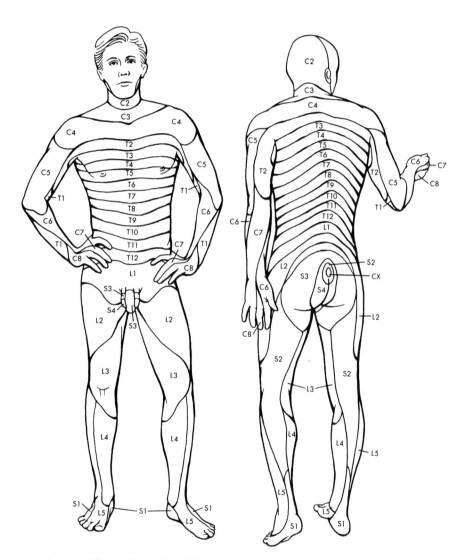

FIG 3-95. Dermatomal map. (From Templin JM: *Anatomy and physiology laboratory manual,* ed 2, St Louis, 1992, Mosby.)

SKELETAL SYSTEM

Skeletal Structure and Bony Landmarks

The following list of bones and skeletal landmarks will assist you in reviewing the skeletal system and bony landmarks of the human body. Following the list of landmarks are several diagrams and illustrations that will help you in locating the landmarks.

I. Skull
   A. Frontal bone
   B. Temporal bone
   C. Parietal bone
   D. Occipital bone
   E. Nasal cavity
   F. Maxilla
   G. Mandible
   H. Zygomatic bone and arch
   I. Mastoid process
   J. Occipital protuberance
   K. Coronal suture
   L. Squamous suture
   M. Lambdoidal suture
   N. Foramen magnum
   O. Styloid process
   P. Sagittal suture
   Q. Orbit
   R. Occipital condyle
   S. Nasal aperture

II. Vertebral column
   A. Vertebral body
   B. Transverse process
   C. Spinous process
   D. Lamina
   E. Pedicle
   F. Vertebral foramen
   G. Superior articular facet
   H. Inferior articular facet
   I. Intervertebral disc

III. Sternum
   A. Manubrium
   B. Jugular notch
   C. Clavicular notch
   D. Body
   E. Xiphoid process

IV. Rib
   A. Head
   B. Neck
   C. Body
   D. Articular facets
   E. Sternal end

V. Clavicle
   A. Sternal end (medial)
   B. Acromial end (lateral)
   C. Body

VI. Scapula
   A. Vertebral border (medial)
   B. Axillary border (lateral)
   C. Spine
   D. Acromion
   E. Coracoid process
   F. Superior angle
   G. Inferior angle
   H. Glenoid fossa
   I. Supraspinous fossa
   J. Infraspinous fossa
   K. Subscapular fossa
   L. Scapular notch
   M. Infraglenoid tubercle
   N. Supraglenoid tubercle

VII. Humerus
   A. Head
   B. Anatomical neck
   C. Surgical neck
   D. Greater tubercle
   E. Lesser tubercle
   F. Intertubercular groove (bicipital)
   G. Deltoid tuberosity
   H. Radial groove
   I. Lateral supracondylar ridge
   J. Medial supracondylar ridge
   K. Lateral epicondyle
   L. Medial epicondyle
   M. Radial fossa
   N. Coronoid fossa
   O. Olecranon fossa
   P. Trochlea
   Q. Capitulum

VIII. Radius
   A. Head
   B. Neck
   C. Radial tuberosity
   D. Styloid process

    E.   Anterior oblique line
    F.   Posterior oblique line
    G.   Interosseous border
IX. Ulna
    A.   Olecranon process
    B.   Trochlear (semilunar) notch
    C.   Coronoid process
    D.   Radial notch
    E.   Tuberosity
    F.   Head
    G.   Styloid process
X. Hand
    A.   Carpals
    B.   Scaphoid
    C.   Lunate
    D.   Triquetrum
    E.   Pisiform
    F.   Trapezium
    G.   Trapezoid
    H.   Capitate
    I.   Hamate
    J.   Hook of hamate
    K.   Metacarpals
    L.   Phalanges
XI. Pelvis
XII. Ilium
    A.   Iliac crest
    B.   Anterior superior iliac spine
    C.   Posterior superior iliac spine
    D.   Anterior inferior iliac spine
    E.   Posterior inferior iliac spine
    F.   Greater sciatic notch
XIII. Ischium
    A.   Ischial tuberosity
    B.   Ischial spine
    C.   Lesser sciatic notch
    D.   Ramus of ischium
XIV. Pubis
    A.   Pubic symphysis
    B.   Body of pubis
    C.   Superior ramus
    D.   Inferior ramus
XV. Acetabulum
XVI. Obturator foramen
XVII. Sacrum
XVIII. Coccyx
XIX. Femur
    A.   Head
    B.   Neck

    C.   Greater trochanter
    D.   Lesser trochanter
    E.   Intertrochanteric line
    F.   Fovea capitis
    G.   Pectineal line
    H.   Linea aspera
    I.   Gluteal tuberosity
    J.   Adductor tubercle
    K.   Medial supracondylar ridge
    L.   Lateral supracondylar ridge
    M.   Medial condyle
    N.   Lateral condyle
    O.   Popliteal surface
    P.   Patellar groove
    Q.   Medial epicondyle
    R.   Lateral epicondyle
    S.   Intercondylar notch
XX. Patella
    A.   Anterior surface
    B.   Posterior surface
    C.   Medial facet
    D.   Lateral facet
XXI. Tibia
    A.   Intercondylar eminence
    B.   Medial condyle
    C.   Lateral condyle
    D.   Tibial tuberosity
    E.   Soleal line
    F.   Interosseous border
    G.   Shaft
    H.   Medial malleolus
XXII. Fibula
    A.   Head
    B.   Styloid process
    C.   Neck
    D.   Interosseous border
    E.   Shaft
    F.   Lateral malleolus
XXIII. Foot
XXIV. Tarsals
    A.   Calcaneus
    B.   Talus
    C.   Navicular bone
    D.   Cuboid
    E.   First cuneiform
    F.   Second cuneiform
    G.   Third cuneiform
    H.   Metatarsals
    I.   Phalanges

Use the following illustrations and drawings (Figs. 3-96 through 3-112) to locate the skeletal landmarks listed on the previous pages.

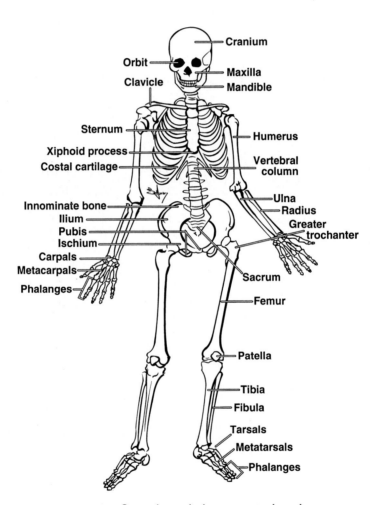

FIG 3-96.   Complete skeleton, anterior view.

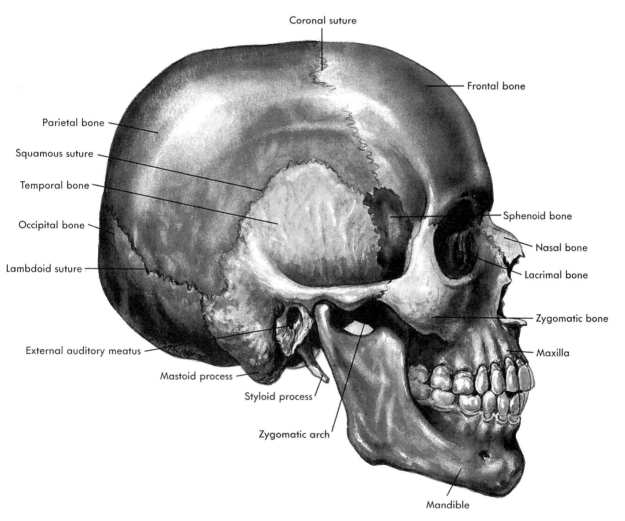

FIG 3-97. Skull viewed from the right side. (Courtesy David J. Mascaro & Associates.)

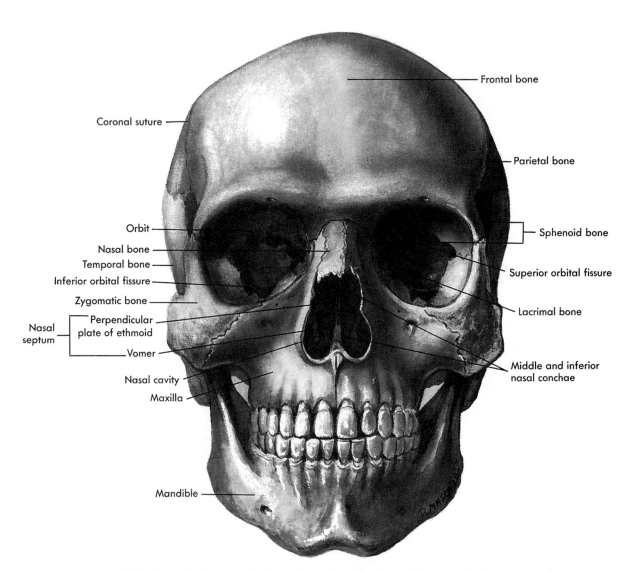

FIG 3-98. Skull, frontal view. (Courtesy David J. Mascaro & Associates.)

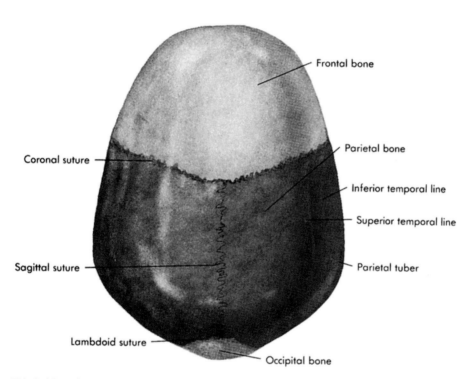

FIG 3-99.   Skull, superior view. (Courtesy David J. Mascaro & Associates.)

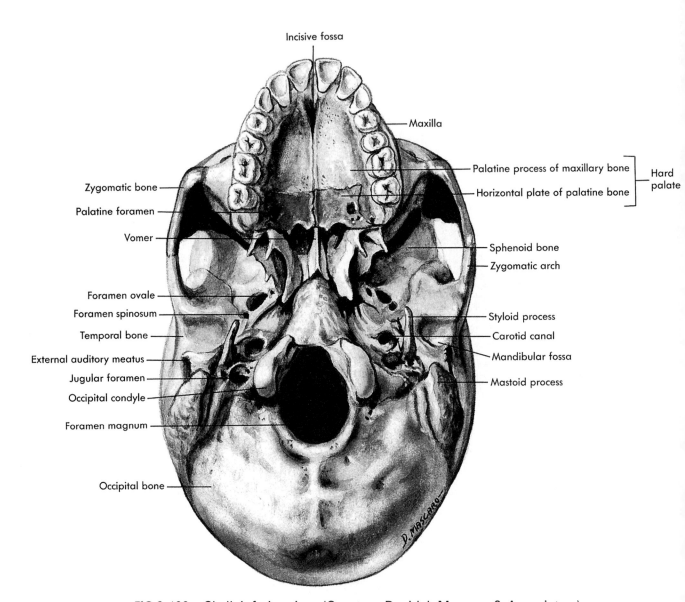

Incisive fossa

Maxilla

Palatine process of maxillary bone

Horizontal plate of palatine bone

Hard palate

Zygomatic bone

Palatine foramen

Vomer

Sphenoid bone

Zygomatic arch

Foramen ovale

Foramen spinosum

Temporal bone

External auditory meatus

Jugular foramen

Occipital condyle

Foramen magnum

Styloid process

Carotid canal

Mandibular fossa

Mastoid process

Occipital bone

FIG 3-100. Skull, inferior view. (Courtesy David J. Mascaro & Associates.)

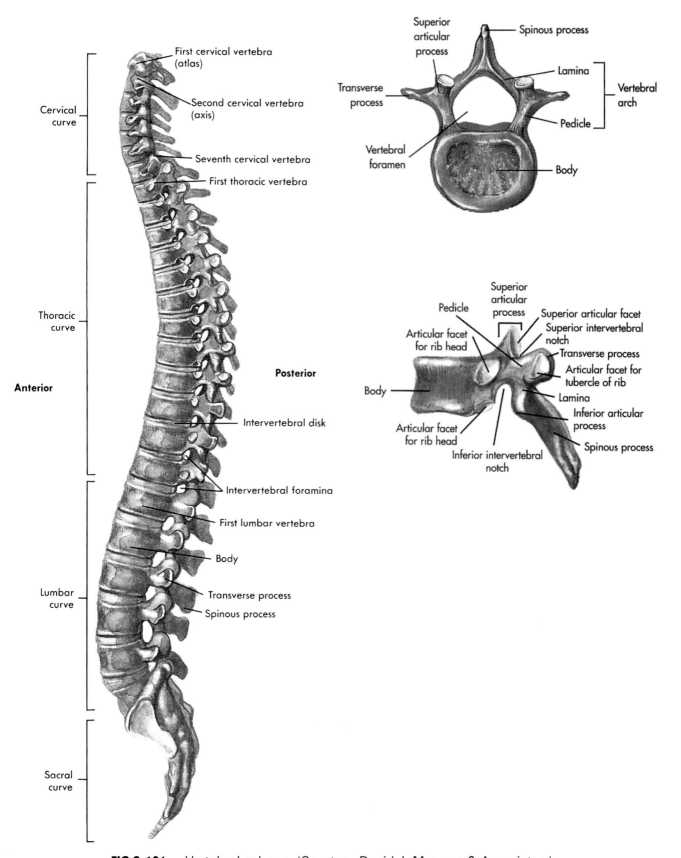

FIG 3-101.   Vertebral column. (Courtesy David J. Mascaro & Associates.)

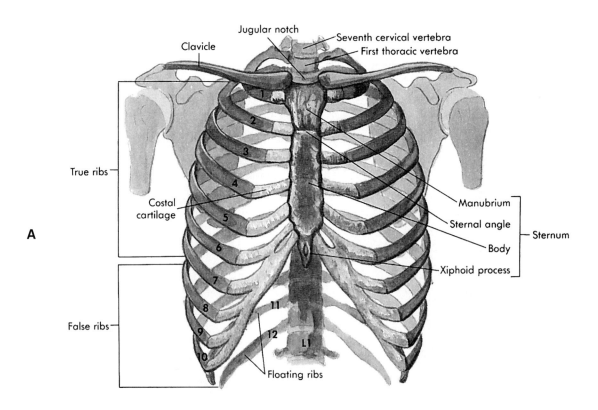

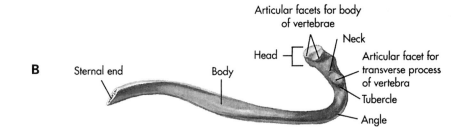

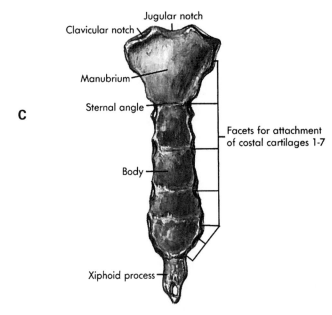

FIG 3-102.   Rib cage **(A)**, typical rib **(B)**, and sternum **(C)**. (Courtesy David J. Mascaro & Associates.)

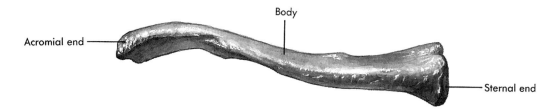

FIG 3-103. Clavicle. (Courtesy David J. Mascaro & Associates.)

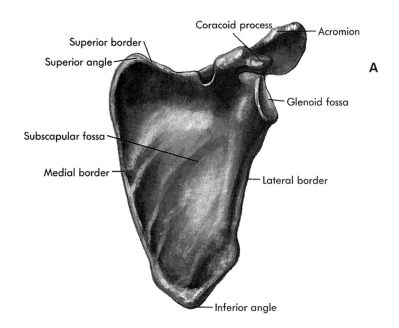

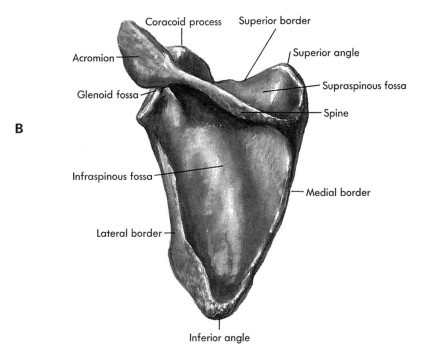

FIG 3-104. Scapula. **A,** Left scapula, anterior view. **B,** Left scapula, posterior view. (Courtesy David J. Mascaro & Associates.)

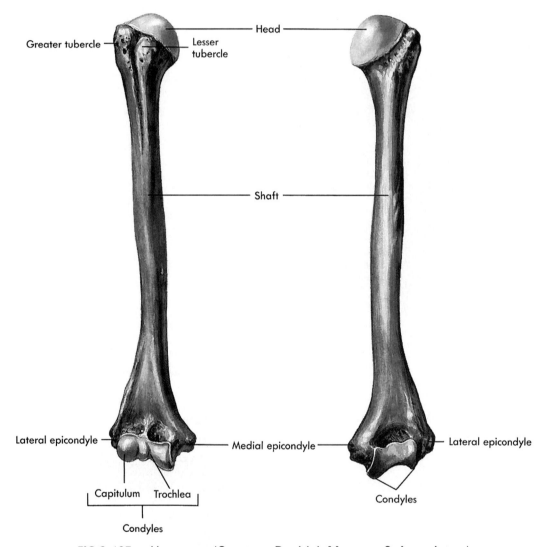

Greater tubercle

Head

Lesser tubercle

Shaft

Lateral epicondyle

Medial epicondyle

Lateral epicondyle

Capitulum   Trochlea

Condyles

Condyles

FIG 3-105.   Humerus. (Courtesy David J. Mascaro & Associates.)

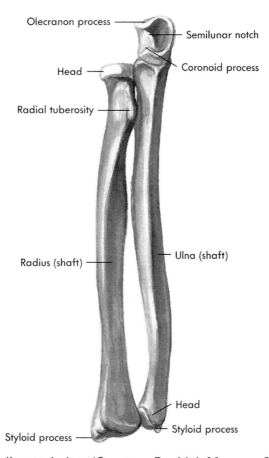

FIG 3-106. Radius and ulna. (Courtesy David J. Mascaro & Associates.)

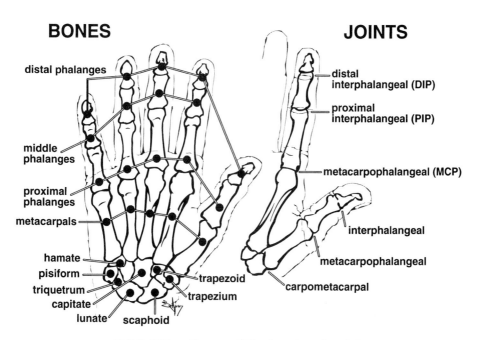

FIG 3-107. Bones of the hand and wrist.

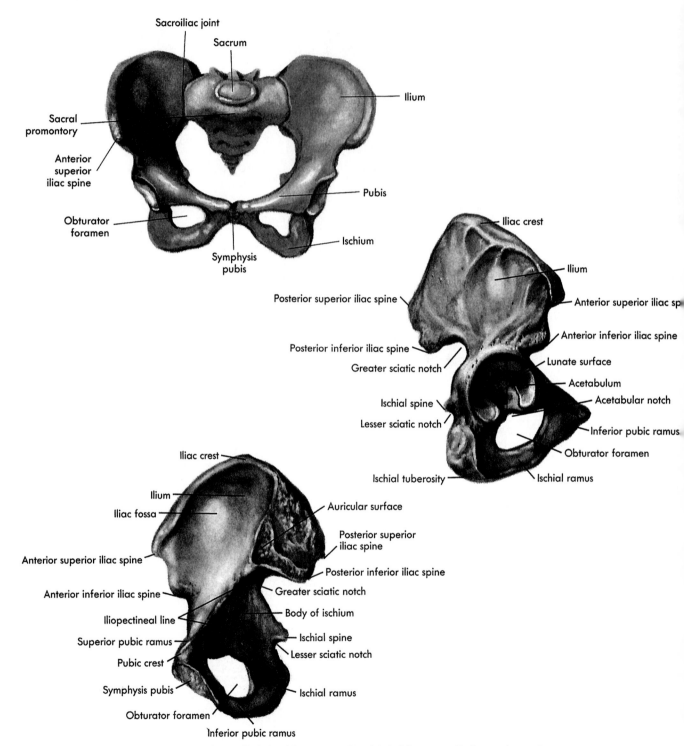

Sacroiliac joint

Sacrum

Ilium

Sacral promontory

Anterior superior iliac spine

Obturator foramen

Pubis

Ischium

Symphysis pubis

Iliac crest

Ilium

Posterior superior iliac spine

Anterior superior iliac sp

Anterior inferior iliac spine

Posterior inferior iliac spine

Lunate surface

Greater sciatic notch

Acetabulum

Acetabular notch

Ischial spine

Lesser sciatic notch

Inferior pubic ramus

Obturator foramen

Ischial tuberosity

Ischial ramus

Iliac crest

Ilium

Iliac fossa

Auricular surface

Posterior superior iliac spine

Anterior superior iliac spine

Posterior inferior iliac spine

Anterior inferior iliac spine

Greater sciatic notch

Iliopectineal line

Body of ischium

Superior pubic ramus

Ischial spine

Pubic crest

Lesser sciatic notch

Symphysis pubis

Ischial ramus

Obturator foramen

Inferior pubic ramus

FIG 3-108. Pelvis. (Courtesy David J. Mascaro & Associates.)

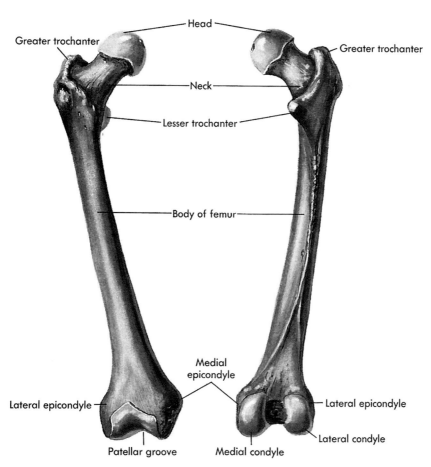

FIG 3-109.   Femur. (Courtesy David J. Mascaro & Associates.)

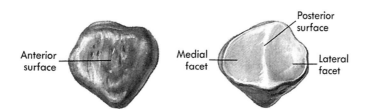

FIG 3-110.   Patella. (Courtesy David J. Mascaro & Associates.)

FIG 3-111. Tibia and fibula.
(Courtesy David J. Mascaro & Associates.)

Lateral condyle

Medial condyle

Head

Tibial tuberosity

Tibia

Fibula

Medial malleolus

Lateral malleolus

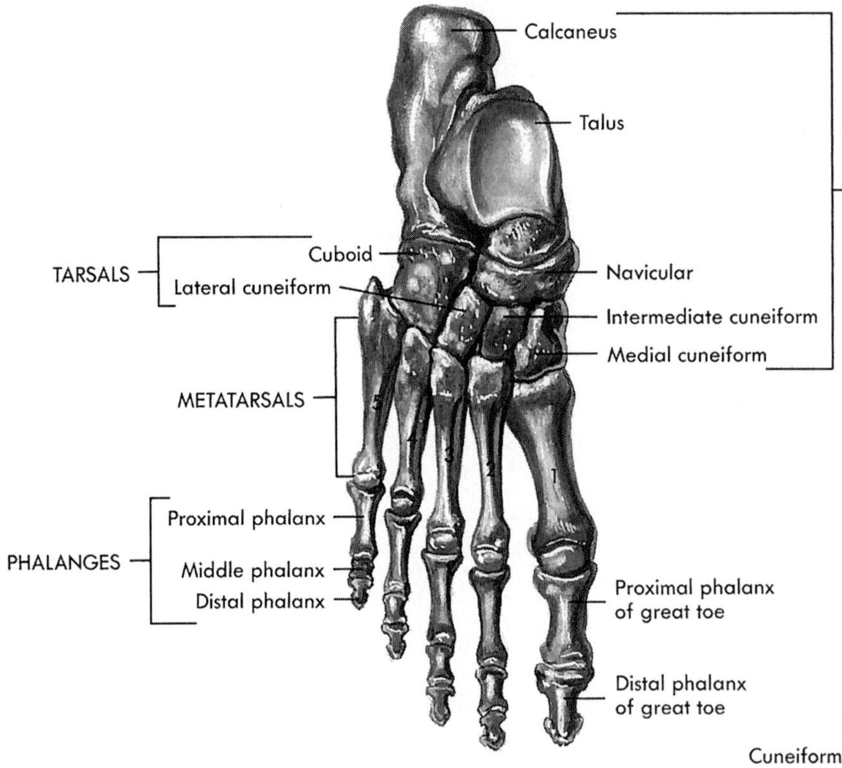

Calcaneus

Talus

TARSALS

Cuboid

Navicular

Lateral cuneiform

Intermediate cuneiform

TARSALS

Medial cuneiform

METATARSALS

Proximal phalanx

Middle phalanx

Distal phalanx

Proximal phalanx
of great toe

PHALANGES

Distal phalanx
of great toe

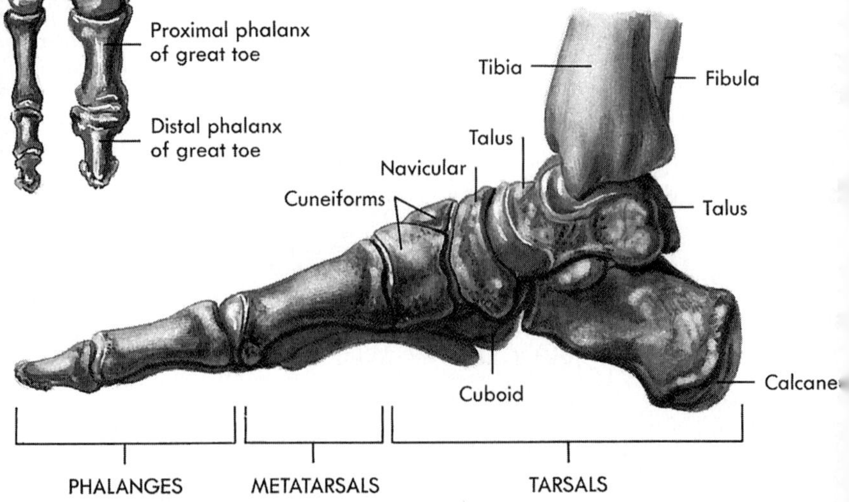

Tibia

Fibula

Talus

Navicular

Talus

Cuneiforms

Cuboid

Calcane

PHALANGES

METATARSALS

TARSALS

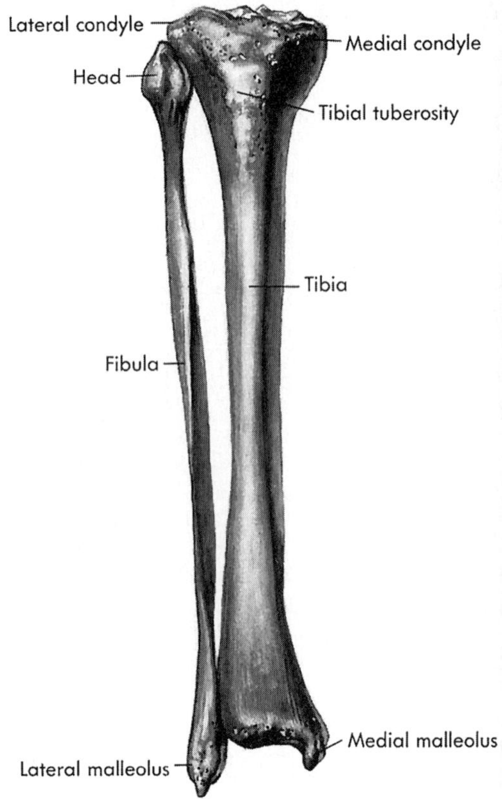

FIG 3-112. Bones of the foot and ankle. (Courtesy David J. Mascaro & Associates.)

CARDIOVASCULAR SYSTEM

Structure

Blood vessels

I. Blood flows from the heart through elastic arteries, muscular arteries, and arterioles to the capillaries.

II. Capillaries are surrounded by loose connective tissue, the adventitia.

III. Capillaries are divided into three types:
  A. Fenestrated capillaries
  B. Sinusoidal capillaries
  C. Continuous capillaries

IV. Blood passes from arterioles through metarterioles and then through the capillary network. The capillary network is drained by venules.

Arteries and veins

I. Except for capillaries and venules, blood vessels have three layers:
  A. *Inner tunica intima:* consists of endothelium, basement membrane, and internal elastic lamina.
  B. *Tunica media (middle layer):* contains circular smooth muscle and elastic fibers.
  C. *Outer tunica adventitia:* is connective tissue.

II. Valves prevent the backflow of blood in the veins.

III. Arteriovenous anastomoses allow blood to flow from arteries to veins without passing through the capillaries. They function in temperature regulation.

Nerve supply

The smooth muscle of the tunica media is supplied by sympathetic nerve fibers.

Aging of the arteries

Arteriosclerosis results from a loss of elasticity in the arteries.

Pulmonary Circulation

The pulmonary circulation moves blood to and from the lungs. The pulmonary trunk arises from the right ventricle and divides to form the pulmonary arteries, which project to the lungs. From the lungs the pulmonary veins return to the left atrium.

Systemic Circulation: Arteries

Aorta

The aorta leaves the left ventricle to form the ascending aorta, aortic arch, and descending aorta (consisting of the thoracic and abdominal aorta).

Coronary arteries

Coronary arteries supply the heart.

Arteries to the head and neck

I.   The brachiocephalic, left common carotid, and left subclavian arteries branch from the aortic arch to supply the head and upper limbs.

II. The common carotid arteries and the vertebral arteries supply the head.

Arteries of the upper limbs

I.   The left subclavian artery continues as the axillary artery and then as the brachial artery. The brachial artery divides into the radial and ulnar arteries.

II. The radial artery supplies the deep palmar arch, and the ulnar artery supplies the superficial palmar arch.

Thoracic aorta and its branches

The thoracic aorta supplies the thoracic organs and the thoracic wall.

Abdominal aorta

The abdominal aorta supplies the abdominal organs and the abdominal wall.

Arteries of the pelvis

The common iliac arteries supply the pelvic organs, pelvic wall, and genitalia.

Arteries of the lower limbs

The lower limbs are supplied by the external iliac arteries, femoral artery, and posterior tibial artery (Fig. 3-113).

Systemic Circulation: Veins

I.   The three major veins returning blood to the heart are:
  A.   Superior vena cava—head, neck, thorax, and upper limbs
  B.   Inferior vena cava—abdomen, pelvis, and lower limbs
  C.   Coronary sinus—heart

II. Veins are of three types:
  A.   Superficial
  B.   Deep
  C.   Sinuses

Coronary veins

Coronary veins enter the coronary sinus or the right atrium and drain the heart.

Veins of the head and neck

I.   The internal jugular veins drain the venous sinuses of the anterior head and neck.

II. The external jugular veins and the vertebral veins drain the posterior head and neck.

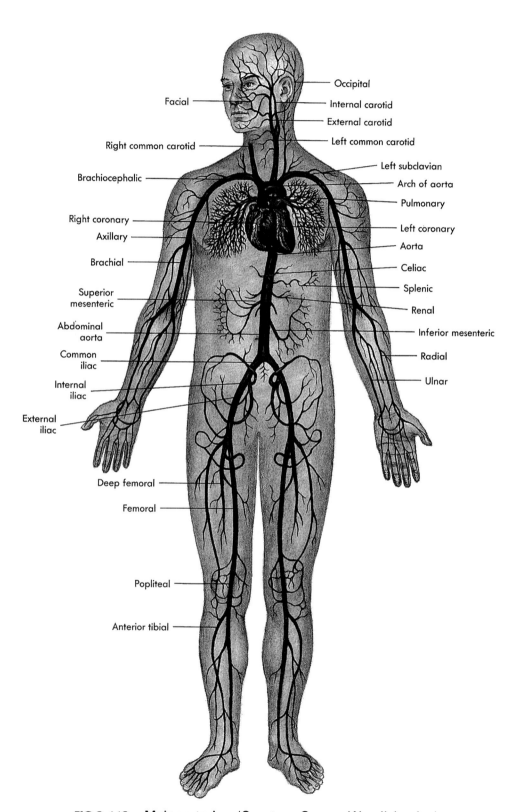

FIG 3-113. Major arteries. (Courtesy George Wassilchenko.)

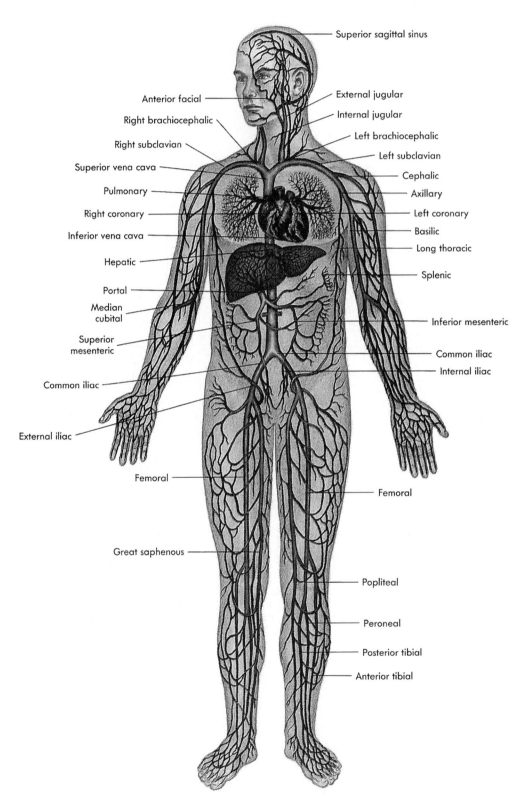

Superior sagittal sinus

Anterior facial

Right brachiocephalic

Right subclavian

Superior vena cava

Pulmonary

Right coronary

Inferior vena cava

Hepatic

Portal

Median cubital

Superior mesenteric

Common iliac

External iliac

Femoral

Great saphenous

External jugular

Internal jugular

Left brachiocephalic

Left subclavian

Cephalic

Axillary

Left coronary

Basilic

Long thoracic

Splenic

Inferior mesenteric

Common iliac

Internal iliac

Femoral

Popliteal

Peroneal

Posterior tibial

Anterior tibial

FIG 3-114. Major veins. (Courtesy George Wassilchenko.)

Veins of the upper limbs

I.   The deep veins are the small ulnar and radial veins of the forearm, which join the brachial vein. The brachial vein drains into the axillary vein.
II. The superficial veins are the basilic, cephalic, and median cubital veins.

Veins of the thorax

The left and right brachiocephalic veins and the azygos veins return blood to the superior vena cava.

Veins of the abdomen and pelvis

Abdominal veins supply the abdomen. They branch into the hepatic (liver) veins.

Veins of the lower limbs

I.   The deep veins are the peroneal, anterior and posterior tibialis, popliteal, femoral, and external iliac veins (Fig. 3-114).
II. The superficial veins are the small and great saphenous veins.

RESPIRATORY SYSTEM

Nose and Nasal Cavity

I.   The bridge of the nose is bone and most of the external nose is cartilage.
II. The openings of the nasal cavity, the external nares, lead to the pharynx.
III. Divisions of the nasal cavity (Fig. 3-115):
    A. *Nasal cavity:* is divided by the nasal septum.
    B. *Anterior vestibule:* contains hairs and traps debris.
    C. *Superior part of the nasal cavity:* contains the olfactory epithelium.

Pharynx

I.   The nasopharynx joins the nasal cavity through the internal nares and contains the internal nares and the openings to the auditory tube and the pharyngeal tonsils.
II. The laryngopharynx opens into the larynx and the esophagus.

Larynx

I.   Cartilage
    A. There are three unpaired cartilages.
    B. There are six paired cartilages. The vocal cords are attached to the arytenoid cartilages.

Trachea

The trachea connects the larynx to the primary bronchi.

Bronchi

The primary bronchi go to each lung. There are primary and secondary bronchi (Fig. 3-116).

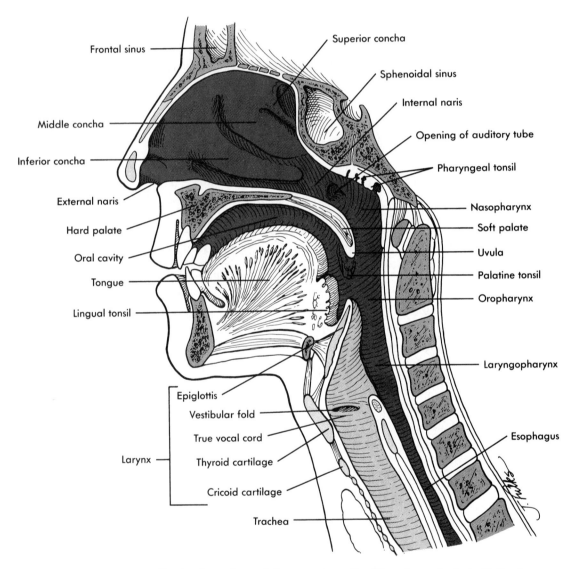

FIG 3-115. Sagittal section of the nasal cavity. (Courtesy Jody L. Fulks.)

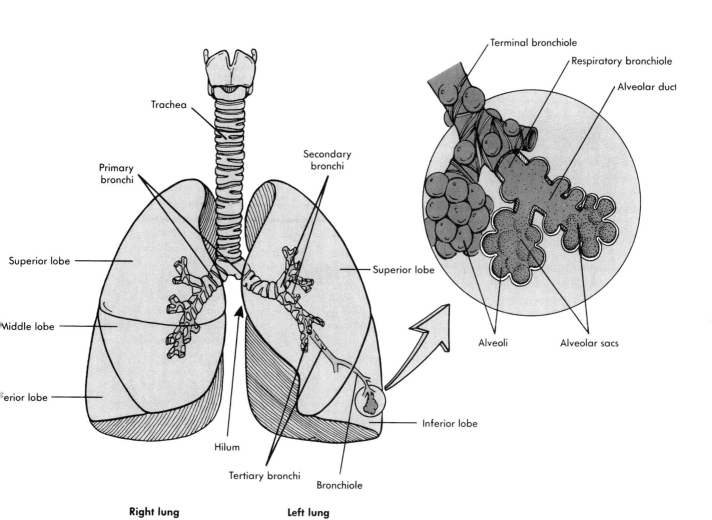

FIG 3-116. Anatomy of the trachea and lungs. (Courtesy Jody L. Fulks.)

Lungs

I.   There are two lungs with several lobes (Fig. 3-117).

II. The airway passages (bronchi) of the lungs branch and decrease in size as they descend into the lungs.

Blood Supply

Deoxygenated blood is transported to the lungs through the pulmonary arteries, and oxygenated blood leaves through the pulmonary veins.

Muscles of Respiration

I.   Contraction of the diaphragm increases thoracic volume.

II. Muscles can elevate the ribs and increase thoracic volume or depress the ribs and decrease thoracic volume.

Nervous Control of Rhythmic Ventilation

I.   The inspiratory center stimulates the muscles of inspiration to contract. Inactivity of the inspiratory center causes passive expiration.

II. The expiratory center stimulates the muscles of forced expiration.

III. The Hering-Breuer reflex inhibits the inspiratory center when the lungs are stretched during inspiration.

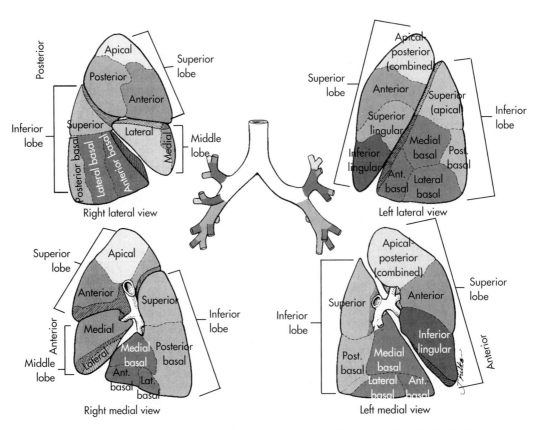

FIG 3-117.   Anatomy of the lobes of the lungs. (Courtesy Jody L. Fulks.)

BASIC PHYSIOLOGY

Energy Systems

I. ATP or phosphagen system
   A. This system is used for adenosine triphosphate (ATP) production during high-intensity, short-duration exercises (e.g., sprinting 150 meters).
   B. This system is the fastest source of ATP available for use by muscles.

II. Anaerobic glycolysis or lactic acid system
   A. This system is the major supplier of ATP during high-intensity, short-duration activities (e.g., sprinting 450 or 750 meters).
   B. This system does not require the presence of oxygen.
   C. It uses only carbohydrates (glycogen and glucose).

III. Aerobic metabolism
   A. The aerobic system is used mainly during low-intensity, long-duration exercise (e.g., running a marathon).
   B. The oxygen system yields the most ATP.

General Functional Characteristics of Muscle

I. Muscle exhibits contractility (shortens), excitability (responds to stimuli), extensibility (stretches), and elasticity (recoils to resting length).

II. According to the *sliding filament theory*, actin and myosin myofilaments do not change length during contraction of skeletal muscle. Instead, they slide past one another in a way that causes the

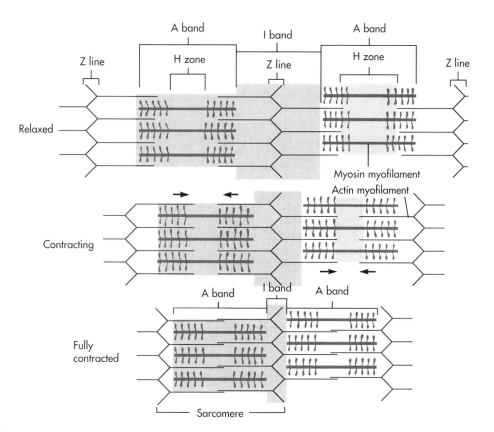

FIG 3-118.   Sliding filament theory—sarcomere shortening. (Courtesy Joan Beck.)

sarcomeres to shorten. During contraction, cross-bridges form between the actin molecules and the heads of the myosin molecules. The cross-bridges form, move, release, and then re-form in a manner similar to the rowing motion of a boat. Movement of the cross-bridges forcefully causes the actin myofilaments at each end of the sarcomere to slide past the myosin myofilaments toward the H zone. As a consequence, the I bands and the H zones become more narrow but the A bands remain constant in length[1] (Fig. 3-118). The H zone may disappear as the actin myofilaments overlap at the center of the sarcomere. As the actin myofilaments slide over the myosin myofilaments, the Z lines are brought closer together and the sarcomere is shortened. The sliding filament theory of muscle contraction includes all of these events.

Skeletal Muscle: Structure

I. Muscle fibers appear striated, are under voluntary control, and are innervated by the somatic nervous system.
II. Muscle fibers are covered by endomysium.
III. Muscle fasciculi, bundles of muscle fibers, are covered by perimysium.
IV. Muscle consisting of fasciculi is covered by epimysium, which in turn is covered by fascia (Fig. 3-119).

Muscle Fibers, Myofibrils, Sarcomeres, and Myofilaments

I. A muscle fiber is a single cell consisting of a cell membrane (sarcolemma), cytoplasm, several nuclei, and myofibrils (Fig. 3-120).
II. Myofibrils consist of many adjoining sarcomeres.
   A. Sarcomeres are bound by Z lines that hold actin myofilaments.
   B. Six actin myofilaments (thin filaments) surround a myosin myofilament (thick filament).
   C. Myofibrils appear striated because of A bands and I bands.
III. A cross-bridge is formed between actin and myosin when the myosin binds to actin.

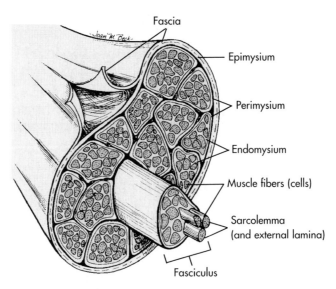

FIG 3-119. Muscle fibers, fasciculi, and their connective tissues. (Courtesy Joan Beck.)

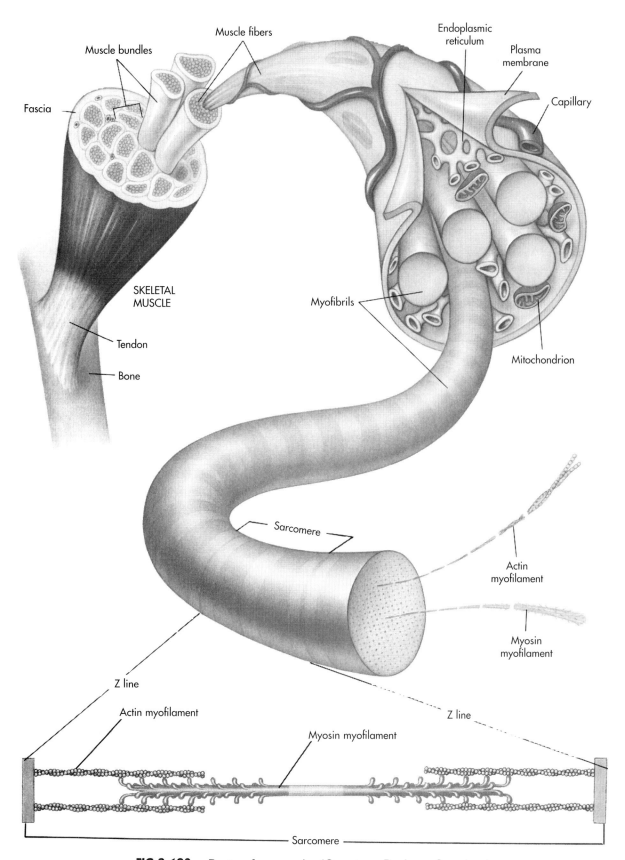

FIG 3-120.   Parts of a muscle. (Courtesy Barbara Cousins.)

KINESIOLOGY

Plane Classification

The study of the joints of the body and their various movements is simplified if we visualize the body as having a series of planes in which these movements occur. Three planes can be used to describe these movements (Fig. 3-121).

I. *Frontal plane:* Divides the body into front and back sections. Movements of the frontal plane:
   A. Abduction-adduction
   B. Radial-ulnar deviation
   C. Eversion-inversion
II. *Sagittal plane:* Divides the body into right and left sections. Movements of the sagittal plane:
   A. Flexion-extension
III. *Horizontal plane (transverse):* Divides the body into upper and lower sections. Movements of the horizontal plane:
   A. Internal-external rotation
   B. Supination-pronation
   C. Right-left rotation
   D. Horizontal abduction-adduction

Degrees of Freedom Classification

I. One degree of freedom—one axis of movement (e.g., elbow)
II. Two degrees of freedom—two axes of movement (e.g., metacarpophalangeal joint of hand)
III. Three degrees of freedom—three axes of movement (e.g., shoulder or hip)

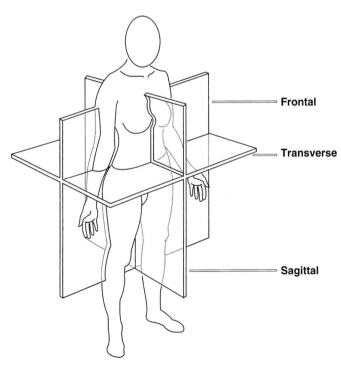

FIG 3-121.   Anatomical planes of motion.

REVIEW QUESTIONS

1. A patient in the anatomical position has:
   a. Heels together
   b. Palms facing anteriorly
   c. Thumbs pointing laterally
   d. Elbow joints extended
   e. All of the above
2. Which of the following terms means "in the direction of the head"?
   a. Cephalad
   b. Cranial
   c. Superior
   d. Cephalic
   e. All of the above
3. The movement known as *circumduction* includes:
   a. Flexion
   b. Extension
   c. Abduction
   d. Adduction
   e. All of the above
4. The axial skeleton includes the:
   a. Femur
   b. Skull
   c. Scapula
   d. Clavicle
   e. All the above
5. Which of the following is classified as a sesamoid bone?
   a. Vertebra
   b. Carpal bone
   c. Patella
   d. Phalanx
   e. Scapula
6. Muscles that steady the proximal part of a limb while movement occurs in the distal part are called:
   a. Prime movers
   b. Antagonists
   c. Synergists
   d. Stabilizers
   e. None of the above
7. The frontal plane:
   a. Divides the body into right and left portions
   b. Divides the body into front and back portions
   c. Divides the body into superior and inferior portions
   d. Is parallel to the midsagittal plane
8. The word *proximal* means:
   a. Farther from the origin of the body part
   b. Above, toward the head
   c. Closer to the origin of the body part
   d. On the outer side of the body

9. The biceps brachii muscle is innervated by the:
    a. Musculocutaneous nerve
    b. Axillary nerve
    c. Ulnar nerve
    d. Median nerve
10. The word *supination* means:
    a. Turning on an axis
    b. Turning the palm up
    c. Turning the palm down
    d. Turning toward the fifth finger side of the hand
11. How many bones are in a normal adult human hand excluding the wrist?
    a. 18
    b. 13
    c. 26
    d. 19
12. Four of the following motions are performed solely by the wrist joint. They are:
    a. Flexion and extension
    b. Supination and pronation
    c. Ulnar and radial deviation
    d. Pronation and flexion
    e. a and d
    f. a and c
13. When you are standing in the anatomical position, the ceiling is:
    a. In the frontal plane
    b. In the sagittal plane
    c. In the horizontal plane
    d. In the vertical plane
14. When you are standing in the anatomical position, the wall you are facing is:
    a. In the frontal plane
    b. In the sagittal plane
    c. In the horizontal plane
    d. In the vertical plane
15. A ligament attaches:
    a. Muscle to bone
    b. Muscle to muscle
    c. Bone to bone
    d. Muscle to tendon
16. The average measurement of elbow flexion is:
    a. 0 to 90 degrees
    b. 0 to 100 degrees
    c. 0 to 135 degrees
    d. None of the above
17. Muscles that perform adduction of the fingers are called:
    a. Adductor pollicis
    b. Dorsal interossei
    c. Palmar interossei
    d. Lumbrical muscles

18. Inversion of the ankle is a combination of two movements. They are:
    a. Supination and adduction
    b. Supination and abduction
    c. Pronation and adduction
    d. Pronation and abduction
19. Which of the following muscles abducts the shoulder?
    a. Posterior deltoid
    b. Serratus anterior
    c. Middle deltoid
    d. Pectoralis major
20. Which of the following muscles is part of the quadriceps femoris muscle group?
    a. Semitendinosus
    b. Biceps femoris
    c. Biceps brachii
    d. Rectus femoris
21. The lateral movement of the scapula is:
    a. Retraction
    b. Abduction
    c. Protraction
    d. Downward rotation
    e. b and c
22. The shoulder girdle has movements of its own. They occur at which of the following joints?
    a. Glenohumeral
    b. Sternoclavicular
    c. Acromioclavicular
    d. b and c
    e. a and b
23. When the sternocleidomastoid muscle contracts bilaterally, it performs:
    a. Lateral flexion
    b. Forward flexion
    c. Extension
    d. Rotation
24. Specific terms are used to describe directional aspects of the body. Regardless of the patient's current position, these terms are always described as if the body were in which position?
    a. Anatomical position
    b. Supine position
    c. Functional position
    d. Dorsal position
25. *Dorsal* is a synonym for:
    a. Posterior
    b. Cranial
    c. Anterior
    d. Ventral
26. The opposite of *cephalad* is:
    a. Ventral
    b. Dorsal
    c. Caudal
    d. Superior
    e. Cranial

27. The xiphoid process is part of the:
    a. Clavicle
    b. Femur
    c. Vertebrae
    d. Sternum
    e. Ulna
28. The muscle that retracts and elevates the scapula is the:
    a. Rhomboid muscle
    b. Thoracospinalis
    c. Pectoralis major
    d. Levator costarum
    e. Latissimus dorsi
29. The muscle that separates the thoracic and abdominal cavities is the:
    a. Psoas major
    b. Psoas minor
    c. Diaphragm
    d. Pectoralis major
30. A patient has a loss of strength at the L1, L2, and L4 levels. Which muscle would you test to confirm this weakness?
    a. Extensor hallucis longus
    b. Quadriceps femoris
    c. Sartorius
    d. Rectus abdominis
31. A patient is complaining of loss of sensation in the deltoid area of the lateral arm. Which nerve would you test to detect the loss of sensation?
    a. C2
    b. C4
    c. T2
    d. C5
32. You ask a patient to abduct the arm. This motion will occur in which plane of motion?
    a. Frontal plane
    b. Sagittal plane
    c. Horizontal plane
    d. a and b
33. A patient complains of pain with supination and pronation. This pain will occur in which plane of motion?
    a. Frontal plane
    b. Sagittal plane
    c. Horizontal plane
    d. Oblique plane
34. The shoulder joint is classified as a ball-and-socket joint. How many degrees of freedom does the shoulder joint have?
    a. 1
    b. 2
    c. 3
    d. 4

35. In a kinesiological study of the hand, the metacarpophalangeal joint has how many degrees of freedom?
    a. 1
    b. 2
    c. 3
    d. 4
36. What is the maximum number of degrees of freedom a single joint can have?
    a. 5
    b. 6
    c. 3
    d. 4
37. Which of the following joint(s) are examples of concave-convex joint relationships?
    a. Glenohumeral joint
    b. Humeroulnar joint
    c. Carpometacarpal joint of thumb
    d. a and b
38. If a muscle elongates over two or more joints at the same time, it will not allow further motion by the agonist because it reaches:
    a. Passive insufficiency
    b. Active insufficiency
    c. Eccentric contraction
    d. Passive tension
39. Which of the following muscles opens the jaw?
    a. Buccinator
    b. Temporalis
    c. Pterygoid medialis
    d. Pterygoid lateralis
40. The origin of the teres major muscle is the:
    a. Midshaft of the humerus
    b. Greater tubercle of the humerus
    c. Lesser tubercle of the humerus
    d. Lateral border of the scapula
41. The insertion of the infraspinatus muscle is the:
    a. Midshaft of the humerus
    b. Lesser tubercle of the humerus
    c. Greater tubercle of the humerus
    d. Bicipital groove
42. Which of the following carpal bones is *not* located on the proximal row?
    a. Lunate
    b. Scaphoid
    c. Trapezium
    d. Triquetrum
    e. Pisiform
43. The origin of the muscle for which the insertion is the lesser tubercle of the humerus is the:
    a. Infraspinous fossa of the scapula
    b. Acromium of the scapula
    c. Supraspinous fossa of the scapula
    d. Subscapular fossa of the scapula

44. The annular ligament is located at the:
    a. Wrist
    b. Shoulder
    c. Elbow
    d. Proximal radioulnar joint

45. Which of the following is an example of a condyloid joint?
    a. Glenohumeral
    b. Sternoclavicular
    c. Proximal interphalangeal
    d. Radiocarpal
    e. Elbow

46. Which of the following motions is performed by the latissimus dorsi muscle in the frontal plane?
    a. Flexion of the shoulder
    b. Extension of the shoulder
    c. Adduction of the shoulder
    d. Internal rotation of the shoulder

47. In the fundamental position, the palms:
    a. Face forward
    b. Face the sides of the body
    c. Face posteriorly
    d. None of the above

48. The temporomandibular joint is elevated by which muscle(s)?
    a. Temporalis
    b. Suprahyoid
    c. Longus coli
    d. Masseter
    e. a and d

49. The scapula is inferiorly rotated by which muscle?
    a. Serratus anterior
    b. Pectoralis major
    c. Levator scapulae
    d. None of the above

50. A 65-year-old patient is having difficulty abducting the hip. Which muscle needs to be strengthened?
    a. Iliopsoas
    b. Tensor fasciae
    c. Gluteus medius
    d. Piriformis

51. Which of the following is *not* a hamstring?
    a. Semimembranosus
    b. Biceps femoris
    c. Rectus femoris
    d. Vastus lateralis
    e. c and d

52. The suprascapular nerve innervates the:
    a. Teres major
    b. Supraspinatus
    c. Infraspinatus
    d. Serratus anterior
    e. b and c

53. Paralysis of spinal cord segments L2, L3, and L4 would be evident in a muscle test of which muscle(s)?
    a. Gluteus medius
    b. Semitendinosus
    c. Gracilis
    d. Sartorius
    e. c and d

54. A patient is having difficulty turning the palm toward the ceiling. At which spinal level would you expect the patient to be injured?
    a. C7-8
    b. C5-6
    c. C2-3
    d. C4-5

55. A 57-year-old male patient is complaining of numbness at the nipple line. What dermatome level would you expect to be involved?
    a. C8
    b. T2
    c. T4
    d. T1

56. A 34-year-old female patient is complaining of numbness in the left medial buttock area. This symptom would be evidence of involvement at which spinal level?
    a. L2
    b. L3
    c. S1
    d. L4

57. If a patient has nerve damage to the L3 dermatome area, where would you expect to find numbness?
    a. Lateral thigh
    b. Lower abdomen
    c. Anteromedial thigh
    d. First and second toe

58. The deltoid ligament adds stability to the:
    a. Elbow joint
    b. Shoulder joint
    c. Ankle joint
    d. Hip joint

59. The ligament that guards against forward displacement of the tibia on the femur is the:
    a. Posterior cruciate ligament
    b. Transverse ligament
    c. Anterior cruciate ligament
    d. Medial collateral ligament

60. The ligament that guards against forward sliding of the femur on the tibia is the:
    a. Posterior cruciate ligament
    b. Transverse ligament
    c. Anterior cruciate ligament
    d. Medial collateral ligament
61. The usual number of thoracic vertebrae is:
    a. 12
    b. 10
    c. 14
    d. 8
62. Capillaries are surrounded by loose connective tissue called:
    a. Tunica
    b. Anastomosis
    c. Adventitia
    d. None of the above
63. The aorta leaves the heart via the:
    a. Right atrium
    b. Left atrium
    c. Right ventricle
    d. Left ventricle
64. The head and neck get their blood supply from the:
    a. Brachiocephalic artery
    b. Left common carotid artery
    c. Left subclavian artery
    d. All the above
65. The Hering-Breuer reflex:
    a. Causes coughing during expiration
    b. Causes a baby to jump when frightened
    c. Inhibits the inhibitory center when the lungs are stretched during inspiration
    d. Causes circulation to slow down when the body is exposed to cold temperatures

REFERENCE
1. Seeley RR: *Anatomy and physiology,* ed 2, St Louis, 1992, Mosby.

SUGGESTED READINGS
Anthony CP: *Textbook of anatomy and physiology,* ed 9, St Louis, 1975, Mosby.
Gould JA: *Orthopaedic and sports physical therapy,* ed 2, St Louis, 1994, Mosby.
Moore KL: *Clinically oriented anatomy,* Baltimore, 1987, Williams & Wilkins.
Thompson CW: *Manual of structural kinesiology,* ed 12, St Louis, 1994, Mosby.

EXAMINATION ANSWER KEY

1. e	**20.** d	**39.** c	**58.** c
2. e	**21.** e	**40.** d	**59.** c
3. e	**22.** d	**41.** c	**60.** a
4. b	**23.** b	**42.** c	**61.** a
5. c	**24.** a	**43.** d	**62.** c
6. d	**25.** a	**44.** d	**63.** d
7. b	**26.** c	**45.** d	**64.** d
8. c	**27.** d	**46.** d	**65.** c
9. a	**28.** a	**47.** b	
10. b	**29.** c	**48.** e	
11. d	**30.** c	**49.** c	
12. f	**31.** d	**50.** c	
13. c	**32.** a	**51.** e	
14. a	**33.** c	**52.** e	
15. c	**34.** c	**53.** e	
16. c	**35.** b	**54.** b	
17. c	**36.** c	**55.** c	
18. a	**37.** d	**56.** d	
19. c	**38.** a	**57.** c	

EXAMINATION ANSWER SHEET

1. _____	20. _____	39. _____	58. _____
2. _____	21. _____	40. _____	59. _____
3. _____	22. _____	41. _____	60. _____
4. _____	23. _____	42. _____	61. _____
5. _____	24. _____	43. _____	62. _____
6. _____	25. _____	44. _____	63. _____
7. _____	26. _____	45. _____	64. _____
8. _____	27. _____	46. _____	65. _____
9. _____	28. _____	47. _____	
10. _____	29. _____	48. _____	
11. _____	30. _____	49. _____	
12. _____	31. _____	50. _____	
13. _____	32. _____	51. _____	
14. _____	33. _____	52. _____	
15. _____	34. _____	53. _____	
16. _____	35. _____	54. _____	
17. _____	36. _____	55. _____	
18. _____	37. _____	56. _____	
19. _____	38. _____	57. _____	

EXAMINATION ANSWER SHEET

1. _____

2. _____

3. _____

4. _____

5. _____

6. _____

7. _____

8. _____

9. _____

10. _____

11. _____

12. _____

13. _____

14. _____

15. _____

16. _____

17. _____

18. _____

19. _____

20. _____

21. _____

22. _____

23. _____

24. _____

25. _____

26. _____

27. _____

28. _____

29. _____

30. _____

31. _____

32. _____

33. _____

34. _____

35. _____

36. _____

37. _____

38. _____

39. _____

40. _____

41. _____

42. _____

43. _____

44. _____

45. _____

46. _____

47. _____

48. _____

49. _____

50. _____

51. _____

52. _____

53. _____

54. _____

55. _____

56. _____

57. _____

58. _____

59. _____

60. _____

61. _____

62. _____

63. _____

64. _____

65. _____

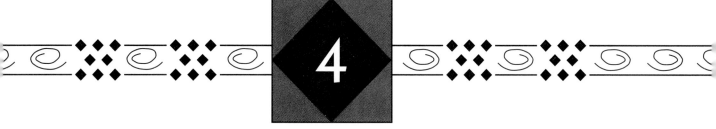

Neuroanatomy and Neurology

The nervous system is the regulatory, controlling, and coordinating system for all the other systems of the human body. It is also the center for all mental activity, including consciousness, memory, and thinking. To perform these functions, the nervous system must collect sensory information from the rest of the body. This information is collected from special sensory nerve endings in the skin, deeper tissues, eyes, ears, and other sensors and transmitted to the spinal cord and brain. The information may be reacted on immediately through a motor response or may be stored and combined with other data in the brain and reacted on at a later time.[1]

The nervous system therefore has three primary functions: (1) collection of sensory information, (2) integration of data (thinking and memory), and (3) motor function (movement). To facilitate the study of the functions and structure of the nervous system, we can subdivide it into two systems: (1) the central nervous system and (2) the peripheral nervous system. Both have distinct features that distinguish them from each other.

The **central nervous system (CNS)** consists of the brain and the spinal cord, both of which are protected by bone. The brain lies within the cranial vault (skull), and the spinal cord is protected by the vertebral canal. The brain joins the spinal canal at the foramen magnum[2] (Fig. 4-1).

The brain is the organ in which the thought processes and memories are integrated and emotions are produced; it is the general control center

for the body. The brain and spinal cord are delicate structures and therefore require the protective covering of the skull (cranial bones) and vertebrae, respectively. Underneath the bony covering is an inner covering of membranes called meninges. The meninges consist of three layers: (1) dura mater, (2) arachnoid, and (3) pia mater[2] (Fig. 4-2).

The brain may be divided into six parts: (1) cerebrum, (2) diencephalon, (3) midbrain, (4) cerebellum, (5) pons, and (6) medulla oblongata (usually called the medulla). At times the terms for the brain can be confusing. The cerebrum is also called the telencephalon. The telencephalon and diencephalon together constitute the prosencephalon or forebrain. The midbrain is also called the mesencephalon. The cerebellum, pons, and medulla all lie in the posterior fossa and together are known as the hindbrain or rhombencephalon (Fig. 4-3).

The spinal cord, which is the downward continuation of the medulla oblongata, has two basic functions: (1) to carry many different nerve pathways to and from the CNS and (2) to coordinate many activities that produce reflexes such as the flexor withdrawal reflex (removal of a body part from a painful stimuli).

The **peripheral nervous system (PNS)** consists of nerves and ganglia outside the vertebral canal. The nerves are groups of axons and their sheaths that run from the CNS to peripheral structures, such as muscles and organs, and from the sensory organs to the CNS.[3] Forty-three pairs of nerves originate in the CNS and make up the PNS. Twelve of the pairs are **cranial nerves,** which originate from the brain; the other 31 pairs are **spinal nerves,** which originate from the spinal cord (8 pairs of cervical nerves, 12 pairs of thoracic nerves, 5 pairs of lumbar nerves, 5 pairs of sacral nerves, and 1 pair of coccygeal nerves). **Ganglia** are nerve cell bodies located outside the CNS.[4]

The PNS has two subdivisions: the **afferent** and **efferent** divisions. The afferent fibers carry sensory impulses to the CNS. The efferent fibers carry motor impulses away from the CNS by cranial or spinal nerves.

The efferent division is further divided into two subdivisions based on the type of effectors supplied. The **somatic nervous system** innervates skeletal muscle and is usually under voluntary control. The **autonomic nervous system** innervates cardiac muscle, smooth muscle, and glands.

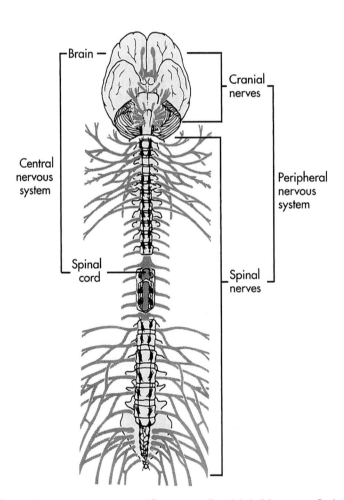

FIG 4-1. Central nervous system. (Courtesy David J. Mascaro & Associates.)

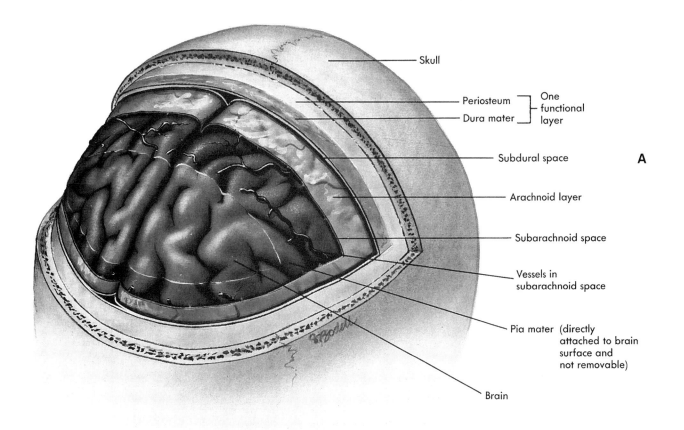

Skull

Periosteum ⎤ One
Dura mater ⎦ functional layer

Subdural space   **A**

Arachnoid layer

Subarachnoid space

Vessels in subarachnoid space

Pia mater (directly attached to brain surface and not removable)

Brain

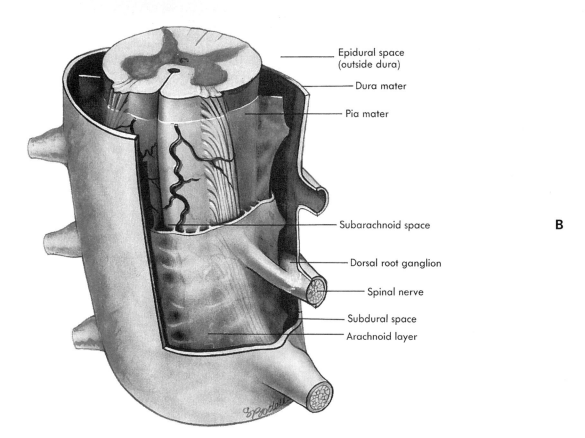

Epidural space (outside dura)

Dura mater

Pia mater

Subarachnoid space   **B**

Dorsal root ganglion

Spinal nerve

Subdural space
Arachnoid layer

FIG 4-2.   Meninges of the brain **(A)** and spinal cord **(B)**. (Courtesy Scott Bodell.)

The primary element of the nervous tissue is the **neuron,** or nerve cell. The nerve cell has three primary components: cell body, dendrites, and axons. The **cell body,** or soma, contains the nucleus, nucleolus, and endoplasmic reticulum. The cell body is the primary location of protein synthesis. **Dendrites** are short, branching extensions of the cell body that receive and conduct electrical impulses toward the cell body. **Axons** are usually a single branch from the cell body and they carry electrical impulses away from the cell body (Fig. 4-4).

There are three basic types of neurons:

1. **Multipolar neurons** have several dendrites and a single axon. (Most motor and CNS neurons are multipolar.)
2. **Bipolar neurons** have a single axon and dendrite (components of sensory organs).
3. **Unipolar neurons** have a single axon. (Most sensory neurons are unipolar.) (Fig. 4-5).

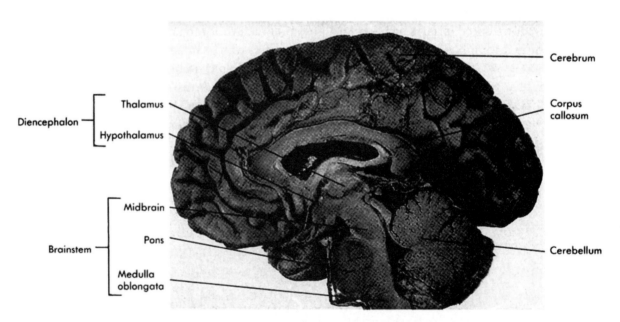

FIG 4-3.   Regions of the brain (midsagittal section). (Courtesy R.T. Hutchings.)

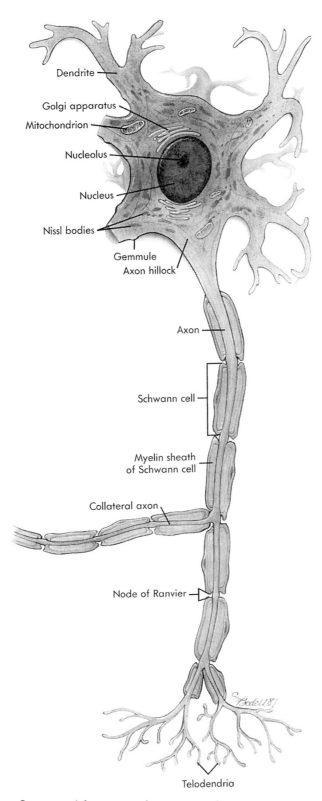

Dendrite

Golgi apparatus

Mitochondrion

Nucleolus

Nucleus

Nissl bodies

Gemmule
Axon hillock

Axon

Schwann cell

Myelin sheath
of Schwann cell

Collateral axon

Node of Ranvier

Telodendria

FIG 4-4. Structural features of neurons. (Courtesy Scott Bodell.)

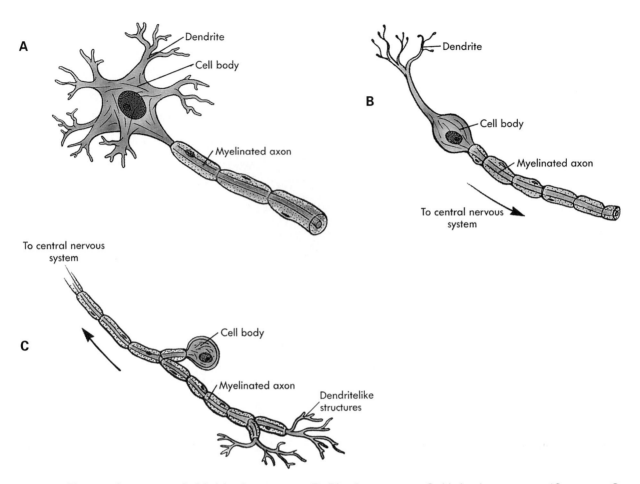

FIG 4-5. Types of neurons. **A,** Multipolar neuron. **B,** Bipolar neuron. **C,** Unipolar neuron. (Courtesy Scott Bodell.)

TERMINOLOGY

Terms	Definitions
1. Central nervous system	Portion of nervous system consisting of the brain and spinal cord (see Fig. 4-1)
2. Peripheral nervous system	Portion of nervous system consisting of nerves and ganglia outside the brain and spinal cord (see Fig. 4-1)

For terms 3-7, see Fig. 4-4

3. Neuron (nerve cell)	Functional unit of the nervous system
4. Dendrite	Branching extension of cell body that brings impulses toward the cell body
5. Axon	Single branch from cell body that takes impulses away from the cell body
6. Nucleolus	Center of axon
7. Myelin	Lipoprotein surrounding some axons; it increases the speed of impulse conduction
8. Synapse	Gap between nerve cells that transmits impulses from one cell to another cell

Terms	**Definitions**
For terms 9-10, see Fig. 4-6	
9. Motor (efferent) neuron	Nerve cell that innervates skeletal, smooth, or cardiac muscle fibers and is multipolar, with its cell body and dendrite in the anterior horn
10. Sensory (afferent) neuron	Nerve cell that arises in skin and runs to the cell body in the dorsal root ganglion
11. Node of Ranvier	Short interval or break in the myelin sheath of a nerve fiber between Schwann cells (see Fig. 4-4)
12. Schwann cell	Cell that forms a myelin sheath around each nerve fiber of the PNS (see Fig. 4-4)
For terms 13-16, see Fig. 4-6	
13. Ventral root	Root of spinal nerve located just outside the spinal cord near the intervertebral foramen; contains efferent (motor) fibers
14. Dorsal root	Root of spinal nerve that contains afferent (sensory) fibers
15. Afferent fibers	Nerve fibers that send impulses from the periphery to the CNS
16. Efferent fibers	Nerve fibers that send impulses from the CNS to the periphery
For terms 17-23, see Fig. 4-3	
17. Cerebrum	Largest and main portion of the brain; it is responsible for the highest mental functions
18. Cerebellum	Posterior portion of the brain attached to the brainstem at the pons; it functions to maintain muscle tone, balance, and coordination of movement
19. Brainstem	Portion of the brain consisting of the midbrain, pons, and medulla oblongata
20. Midbrain	Center for visual reflexes; it is located below the cerebrum
21. Pons	Portion of the brainstem between the medulla oblongata and midbrain; it relays information from the cerebrum to the cerebellum and acts as the sleep and respiratory center
22. Medulla oblongata	Most inferior portion of the brainstem; it is the center for reflexes of regulation of heart rate, coughing, breathing, swallowing, sneezing, vomiting, and blood vessel diameter
23. Corpus callosum	Largest commissure (connection) of the brain connecting the cerebral hemispheres

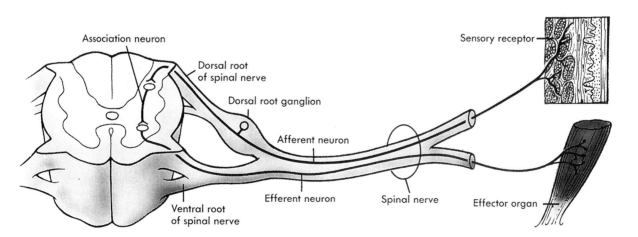

FIG 4-6. Reflex arc, including the sensory receptor, afferent (sensory) neuron, association neuron, efferent (motor) neuron, and effector organ. (Courtesy Scott Bodell.)

Terms	Definitions
For terms 24-27, see Fig. 4-7	
24. Frontal lobe of cerebrum	Lobe located in the anterior portion of the skull; it controls personality, motor movement, and expressive speech
25. Occipital lobe of cerebrum	Lobe located in the posterior portion of the skull; it controls vision and recognition of size, shape, and color
26. Parietal lobe of cerebrum	Lobe located between the frontal and occipital lobes; it controls gross sensation such as touch and pressure as well as fine sensation such as determining texture, weight, size, and shape
27. Temporal lobe of cerebrum	Lobe located under the frontal and parietal lobes; it receives and evaluates olfactory (smelling) and auditory (hearing) information and is the center for behavior and language interpretation
28. Thalamus	Major sensory relay center; it influences mood and movement and is the pain perception center (see Fig. 4-3)
29. Subthalamus	Small area immediately inferior to the thalamus; it contains several nerve tracts that control motor functions
30. Epithalamus	Small area superior and posterior to the thalamus; it contains the habenular nuclei, which have an influence on emotions through the sense of smell, and the pineal body, which is thought to influence the onset of puberty
31. Hypothalamus	Most inferior portion of the diencephalon; it regulates many endocrine functions (i.e., metabolism, reproduction, response to stress, urine production), as well as body temperature, hunger, thirst, satiety, swallowing and emotions (see Fig. 4-3)
32. Satiety	State of complete satisfaction of hunger or thirst
33. Prosencephalon	Embryonic brain structure that becomes the cerebrum in the adult
34. Mesencephalon	Embryonic brain structure that becomes the midbrain in the adult
35. Rhombencephalon	Embryonic brain structure that becomes the pons and cerebellum in the adult; contains nerve pathways, reflex center, muscle coordination, and balance
36. Meninges	Connective tissue layers that surround and protect the brain and spinal cord
For terms 37-40, see Fig. 4-2	
37. Dura mater	Most superficial and thickest layer of the meninges
38. Arachnoid	Very thin second layer of the meninges
39. Subdural space	Space between arachnoid and dura mater
40. Pia mater	Third meningeal layer, which is bound tightly to the surface of the brain and spinal cord
41. Cerebrospinal fluid	Fluid that circulates through the subarachnoid space; it is similar to plasma and acts as a protective cushion
For terms 42-43, see Fig. 4-7	
42. Central sulcus	Groove that separates the frontal and parietal lobes
43. Lateral fissure	Deep fold that separates the temporal lobe from the rest of the cerebrum

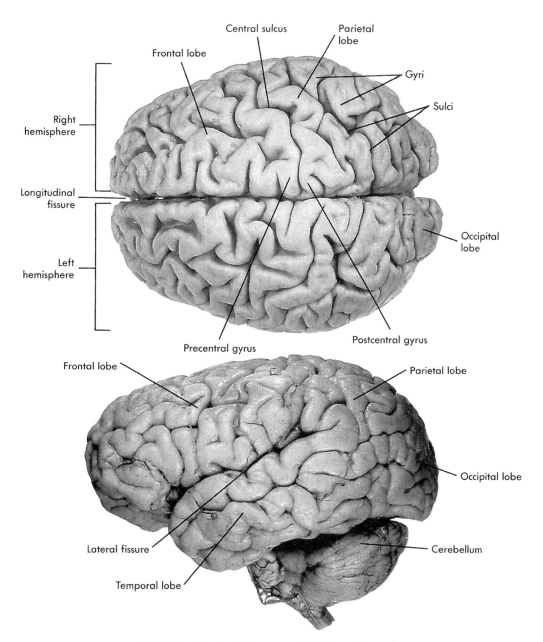

FIG 4-7. Brain. (Courtesy R.T. Hutchings.)

Terms

For terms 44-49, see Fig. 4-8

44. Internal carotid artery
45. Middle cerebral artery

46. Anterior cerebral artery
47. Right and left vertebral arteries

48. Basilar artery

49. Circle of Willis

Definitions

Artery that supplies the anterior part of the brain

Continuation of the internal carotid artery; it supplies the lateral cerebral hemispheres

Artery that supplies the medial surface of the brain

Arteries that run through the neck through the transverse foramen of the cervical vertebrae and then enter the base of the brain through the foramen magnum to supply the posterior brain

Artery that supplies parts of the cerebellum, pons, and midbrain; it branches to form the posterior cerebral arteries

Circle of interconnected anterior and posterior cerebral arteries and internal carotid arteries at the base of the brain; these vessels are joined by the posterior and anterior communicating arteries

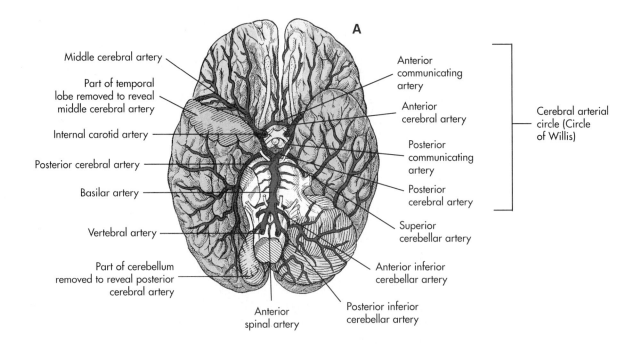

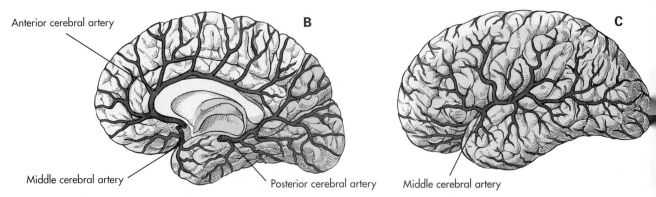

FIG 4-8.   Circulation to the brain. **A,** Inferior view. **B,** Medial view. **C,** Lateral view. (Courtesy Karen Waldo.)

Terms

Definitions

For terms 50-52, see Fig. 4-9

50. Conus medullaris

Cone-shaped region formed by the tapering of the spinal cord; it is located immediately inferior to the lumbar enlargement, and its tip is at L2, the end of the spinal cord

51. Cauda equina

The group of spinal nerves including the conus medullaris and other numerous spinal nerves at the lower end of the spinal cord; they resemble a horse's tail in appearance and are therefore called the cauda equina (Latin for "horse's tail")

52. Filum terminale

Cord of pia mater extending from the conus medullaris inferiorly; it anchors the spinal cord to the coccyx

53. White matter

White matter that is visible on cross section of the spinal cord; it consists of nerve tracts

54. Gray matter

Central gray matter visible on cross section of the spinal cord; it consists of nerve cell bodies and dendrites

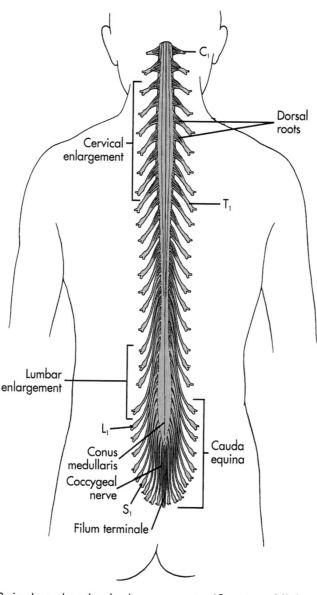

FIG 4-9. Spinal cord and spinal nerve roots. (Courtesy Michael Schenk.)

Terms	**Definitions**
55. Funiculus	Subdivision or column of white matter in the spinal cord; in each half of the spinal cord the white matter is organized into three columns or funiculi (anterior or ventral, posterior or dorsal, and lateral)
56. Fasciculi	Subdivisions or tracts of the funiculus in the white matter made up of small bundles of individual axons that carry impulses to (ascending) and from (descending) the brain
57. Horns	Subdivisions of the central gray matter that resemble a horn in shape
58. Anterior (ventral) horn	Section of spinal cord that contains the cell bodies of the motor neurons
59. Posterior (dorsal) horn	Section of spinal cord that contains the axons of sensory neurons, which synapse with the cell bodies of neurons here
60. Lateral horn	Section of spinal cord that contains the cell bodies of autonomic neurons
61. Reflex	Automatic reaction to stimuli that occurs without conscious thought
62. Stretch reflex	Reflex in which the muscle spindles detect stretch of skeletal muscles and cause the muscle to shorten reflexively
63. Golgi tendon reflex	Reflex in which Golgi tendon organs respond to increased tension within tendons and cause skeletal muscles to relax
64. Flexor withdrawal reflex	Reflex in which the activation of pain receptors causes muscle contraction and the removal of a part of the body from a painful stimulus
65. Upper motor neuron	Neuron located in the cerebral cortex, cerebellum, and brainstem
66. Lower motor neuron	Neuron located in the cranial nuclei or the ventral horn of the spinal cord gray matter
67. Pyramidal system	System of nerve fibers that maintains muscle tone and controls fine, skilled movements
68. Corticospinal tract	Group of nerve fibers that controls muscle movements below the head
69. Corticobulbar tract	Group of nerve fibers that innervates the head muscles
70. Extrapyramidal tract	Group of nerve fibers involved in conscious and unconscious muscle movements, posture, and balance

CRANIAL NERVES (FIG. 4-10)

	Function	
Cranial nerve	**Sensory**	**Motor**
I: Olfactory	Smell	—
II: Optic	Sight	—
III: Oculomotor	—	Eye and eyelid movement
IV: Trochlear	—	Eye movement
V: Trigeminal		
Ophthalmic branch	Sensation from forehead, eye, superior nasal cavity	—
Maxillary branch	Sensation from inferior nasal cavity, face, upper teeth	—
Mandibular branch	Sensation from jaw, lower teeth, and anterior tongue	Mastication
VI: Abducens	—	Eye movement
VII: Facial	Taste	Facial expression
VIII: Vestibulocochlear		
Vestibular branch	Equilibrium	—
Cochlear branch	Hearing	—
IX: Glossopharyngeal	Taste	Swallowing
X: Vagus	Sensation from larynx, trachea, heart, and much of viscera of thorax and abdomen	Movement of various organs
XI: Accessory	—	Movement of neck and shoulders
XII: Hypoglossal	—	Tongue movement

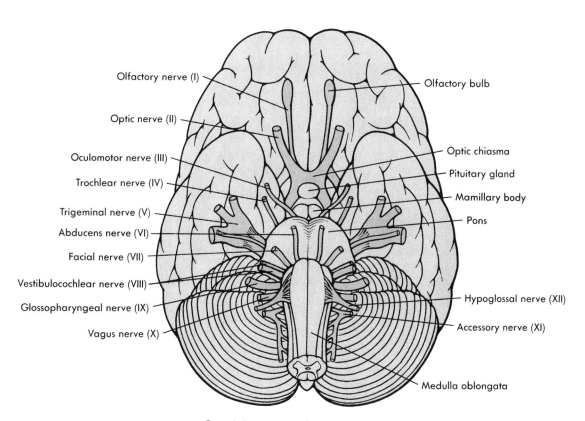

FIG 4-10. Cranial nerves. (Courtesy Michael Schenk.)

SEGMENTAL INNERVATION AND MOTOR RESPONSES

Spinal cord segment	Key movements to test
C4	Shoulder shrug
C5	Shoulder abduction, shoulder external rotation
C6	Elbow flexion, wrist extension
C7	Elbow extension, wrist flexion
C8	Ulnar deviation, thumb and small finger abduction, wrist flexion
T1	Finger approximation
L2	Hip flexion
L3	Knee extension, hip flexion
L4	Knee extension, ankle dorsiflexion
L5	Ankle dorsiflexion, large toe dorsiflexion, ankle eversion
S1	Plantar flexion, plantar eversion, knee flexion
S2	Knee flexion, ankle plantar flexion

SEGMENTAL INNERVATION AND REFLEX TESTING

Nerve/spinal cord segments	Muscle/reflex to test	Stimulus
Cranial nerve V	Jaw jerk	Tap mandible while it is in half-open position
C5-6	Biceps	Tap biceps tendon
C7-8	Triceps brachii	Tap triceps brachii tendon
L3-4	Patellar tendon (knee jerk)	Tap patellar (quadriceps) tendon
S1-2	Achilles tendon	Tap Achilles tendon

SEGMENTAL INNERVATION AND SENSORY RESPONSES

Spinal cord segment	Key segmental sensory areas to test
C6	Thumb and index finger, radial border of hand
C7	Middle three fingers
C8	Ring and small finger, ulnar border of hand
L2	Medial thigh
L3	Anteromedial and distal thigh
L4	Medial aspect of large toe
L5	Web space between large and second toes
S1	Below lateral malleolus, back of heel
S4	Saddle and anal region

SYMPTOMS OF NERVE ROOT SYNDROMES

Compression of a nerve root is usually accompanied by one or more of the following symptoms:
- Pain in the region supplied by the nerve roots
- Radicular loss of sensitivity according to the dermatomes (see Fig. 3-95)
- Motor loss of the muscles innervated by the corresponding roots
- Deep tendon reflex changes

Spinal cord segment(s)	Sensation	Muscle(s) involved	Tendon reflex
Combined C3-4	Pain in shoulder region	Partial or total paralysis of diaphragm	No change
C5	Pain over lateral shoulder (deltoid area)	Disturbance of innervation of deltoid and biceps	Diminished or absent biceps reflex
C6	Pain along dermatome on outer aspect of arm and forearm to thumb	Paralysis of biceps and brachio-radialis	Diminished or absent biceps reflex
C7	Pain along dermatome lateral and dorsal to C6 dermatome including index to ring fingers	Paralysis of triceps brachii and pronator teres	Diminished or absent triceps reflex
C8	Pain along dermatome to C7 extending to little finger	Small muscles of hand atrophy, especially hypothenar eminence	Diminished triceps brachii reflex
L3	Pain along dermatome from greater trochanter to extensor side of thigh	Paralysis of quadriceps	Absent quadriceps reflex (knee jerk)
L4	Pain along dermatome from lateral surface of thigh to anteromedial side of leg plus medial part of sole	Paralysis of quadriceps and tibialis anterior	Diminished quadriceps reflex (knee jerk)
L5	Pain along dermatome from lateral condyle of femur over anterior and outer leg to large toe	Paralysis/atrophy of extensor hallucis longus, and extensor digitorum brevis	Absent tibialis posterior reflex
S1	Pain along dermatome from flexor surface of thigh to outer and posterior side of leg and over lateral malleolus	Paralysis of peroneals and at times triceps surae	Absent triceps surae reflex (ankle jerk)
Combined L4-5	Pain along L4-5 dermatome	Paralysis of all extensor muscles of ankle and weak quadriceps	Diminished quadriceps reflex and absent tibialis posterior reflex
Combined L5-S1	Pain along L5-S1 dermatomes	Paralysis of extensors of toes, peroneals	Absent tibialis posterior and triceps surae reflexes

PARALYSIS DUE TO INJURY TO THE BRANCHES OF THE BRACHIAL PLEXUS (FIGS. 4-11 TO 4-13)

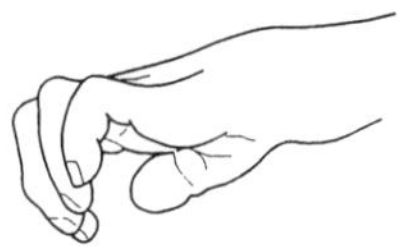

FIG 4-11. Paralysis of the median nerve, resulting in "ape hand." (From Hartley A: *Practical joint assessment: upper quadrant,* ed 2, St Louis, 1995, Mosby.)

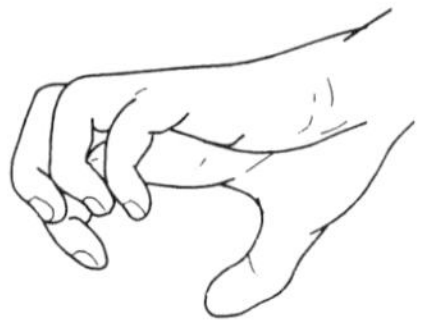

FIG 4-12. Paralysis of the ulnar nerve, resulting in "claw hand." (From Hartley A: *Practical joint assessment: upper quadrant,* ed 2, St Louis, 1995, Mosby.)

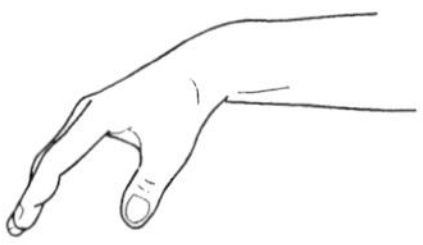

FIG 4-13. Paralysis of the radial nerve, resulting in "drop wrist." (From Hartley A: *Practical joint assessment: upper quadrant,* ed 2, St Louis, 1995, Mosby.)

REVIEW QUESTIONS

1. The median nerve has mainly:
   a. Sensory distribution
   b. Motor distribution
   c. Equal sensory and motor distribution
   d. All the above
2. The largest peripheral nerve in the body is the:
   a. Femoral
   b. Brachial
   c. Musculocutaneous
   d. Sciatic
3. The primary function of cranial nerve II is:
   a. Taste
   b. Smell
   c. Sight
   d. Hearing
4. The function of cranial nerve III is primarily:
   a. Motor
   b. Sensory
   c. Smell
   d. Eye movement
   e. a and d
5. A dendrite:
   a. Is the functional unit of the nervous system
   b. Brings impulses toward the cell body
   c. Takes impulses away from the cell body
   d. Is the gap between nerve cells
6. The area of the cerebrum controlling vision is the:
   a. Frontal lobe
   b. Occipital lobe
   c. Parietal lobe
   d. Temporal lobe
7. The thalamus:
   a. Is the major sensory relay center
   b. Receives and evaluates olfactory and auditory impulses
   c. Contains the habenular nuclei
   d. Controls motor functions
8. The area of the cerebrum that controls expressive speech is the:
   a. Frontal lobe
   b. Occipital lobe
   c. Parietal lobe
   d. Temporal lobe
9. The mesencephalon of the brain:
   a. Becomes the cerebrum
   b. Becomes the midbrain
   c. Is the third meningeal layer of the brain
   d. Becomes the pons

10. The prosencephalon of the brain:
    a. Separates the frontal and parietal lobes
    b. Contains nerve pathways and reflex centers
    c. Is the connective tissue around the brain
    d. Becomes the cerebrum

11. Shoulder shrugs would be a movement to test for which spinal segment?
    a. C3
    b. C4
    c. C5
    d. C6

12. The triceps brachii reflex is a test for which spinal segment(s)?
    a. C5
    b. C6
    c. C7-8
    d. C8-T1

13. A patient injured her back lifting a patient at a nursing home. The patient's chief complaints are pain in the left leg and numbness over the lateral malleolus. The level of involvement is:
    a. L2
    b. L4
    c. L5
    d. S1

14. A patient was involved in a car accident and is complaining of neck pain and numbness in the ring and little fingers. This patient is having an MRI to rule out the possibility of a ruptured disc. What level of nerve impingement would you suspect?
    a. C3
    b. C4
    c. C7
    d. C8

15. The knee reflex or knee jerk is a test for which spinal segments?
    a. L1-2
    b. L2-3
    c. L3-4
    d. L5-S1

16. A patient complaining of pain on the outer aspect of the arm and forearm down to the thumb would be expected to have involvement of spinal segment:
    a. C2
    b. C3
    c. C6
    d. C8

17. Cranial nerve VI is the:
    a. Trigeminal nerve
    b. Abducens nerve
    c. Optic nerve
    d. Oculomotor nerve

18. The motor nerve for the muscles of mastication is the:
    a. Facial nerve
    b. Abducens nerve
    c. Masseter nerve
    d. Trigeminal nerve
19. The cranial nerves are named as well as numbered. Which of the following is correct?
    a. Cranial nerve III is the facial nerve
    b. Cranial nerve IX is the hypoglossal nerve
    c. Cranial nerve X is the vagus nerve
    d. Cranial nerve VI is the trochlear nerve
20. The nerve supply for the muscle that initiates abduction of the shoulder joint (arm) is the:
    a. Long thoracic nerve
    b. Radial nerve
    c. Suprascapular nerve
    d. Axillary nerve
21. The nerve supply for the muscle that inserts into the lesser tubercle of the humerus is the:
    a. Radial nerve
    b. Thoracodorsal nerve
    c. Upper and lower subscapular nerves
    d. Long thoracic nerve
22. The cardiac muscle and smooth muscle are innervated by the:
    a. Somatic nervous system
    b. Autonomic nervous system
    c. Thoracic nervous system
    d. None of the above
23. The portion of the brain responsible for the highest mental functions is the:
    a. Cerebrum
    b. Cerebellum
    c. Brainstem
    d. Midbrain
24. The portion of the brain that is the center for reflexes of regulation of heart rate, coughing, breathing, and swallowing is the:
    a. Pons
    b. Midbrain
    c. Medulla oblongata
    d. Corpus callosum
25. The temporal lobe is separated from the rest of the cerebrum by the:
    a. Central sulcus
    b. Lateral fissure
    c. Subdural space
    d. Medial sulcus
26. Blood is supplied to the anterior part of the brain by the:
    a. Anterior cerebral artery
    b. Posterior cerebral artery
    c. Anterior vertebral artery
    d. Internal carotid artery

27. The end of the spinal cord is at level:
    a. L2
    b. L3
    c. S1
    d. S4

28. A patient complaining of pain in the shoulder over the deltoid area may be experiencing referred pain from:
    a. C3-4
    b. C5
    c. C6
    d. C7

29. The nerve that may be palpated immediately below the head of the fibula is the:
    a. Tibial nerve
    b. Fibula nerve
    c. Common peroneal nerve
    d. Plantaris nerve

REFERENCES

1. Guyton AC: *Basic neuroscience,* Philadelphia, 1987, WB Saunders.
2. Anthony CP: *Anatomy and physiology,* ed 12, St Louis, 1987, Mosby.
3. Seeley RR: *Anatomy and physiology,* ed 2, St Louis, 1992, Mosby.
4. Booher JM: *Athletic injury assessment,* ed 3, St Louis, 1994, Mosby.

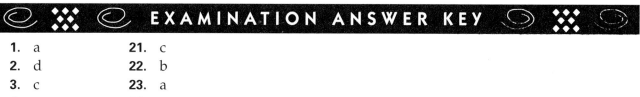

EXAMINATION ANSWER KEY

1.	a	**21.**	c
2.	d	**22.**	b
3.	c	**23.**	a
4.	e	**24.**	c
5.	b	**25.**	b
6.	b	**26.**	d
7.	a	**27.**	a
8.	a	**28.**	b
9.	b	**29.**	c
10.	d		
11.	b		
12.	c		
13.	d		
14.	d		
15.	c		
16.	c		
17.	b		
18.	d		
19.	c		
20.	d		

EXAMINATION ANSWER SHEET

1. _____
2. _____
3. _____
4. _____
5. _____
6. _____
7. _____
8. _____
9. _____
10. _____
11. _____
12. _____
13. _____
14. _____
15. _____
16. _____
17. _____
18. _____
19. _____

20. _____
21. _____
22. _____
23. _____
24. _____
25. _____
26. _____
27. _____
28. _____
29. _____

EXAMINATION ANSWER SHEET

1. _____

2. _____

3. _____

4. _____

5. _____

6. _____

7. _____

8. _____

9. _____

10. _____

11. _____

12. _____

13. _____

14. _____

15. _____

16. _____

17. _____

18. _____

19. _____

20. _____

21. _____

22. _____

23. _____

24. _____

25. _____

26. _____

27. _____

28. _____

29. _____

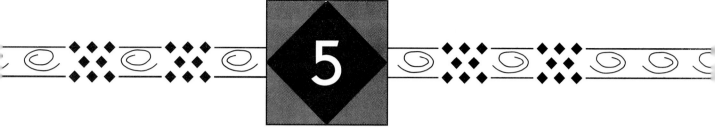

Physical Disabilities

Physical therapist assistants should be able to describe the etiology, pathology, signs, and symptoms of the most prevalent disorders and diseases. In this chapter these disorders are divided into orthopedic, neurological, soft tissue, pulmonary, cardiovascular, and skin disabilities.

Physical therapist assistants also should be able to describe the rationale, objectives, indications, and contraindications of various physical therapy treatments for these disorders. Specific treatment procedures and modalities are discussed in later chapters.

ORTHOPEDIC (MUSCULOSKELETAL) DISORDERS

Musculoskeletal disorders are one of the primary causes of chronic pain and physical handicap in our society because the population is becoming older, more physically fit, and more health conscious.

Diseases of the Bone

I. Osteomyelitis is an inflammation of the bone, especially of the bone marrow. It affects primarily children and adolescents, whose bones are still growing. Long bones are most commonly affected in the area of the growth plate.

II. Tuberculosis of the bone is primarily a disease of the lungs, but the infection can spread to the bones. The ends of long bones are most often affected.
  A. Pott's disease is a form of tuberculosis that affects the vertebral column of children.

III. Diseases of vitamin and mineral deficiencies
  A. Rickets is a disease of infancy and early childhood in which the bones do not properly ossify or harden. It is caused by a vitamin D deficiency. Vitamin D is necessary for the absorption of calcium and phosphorus.
  B. Osteomalacia is similar to rickets, but it is a softening or decalcification of the bones of adults. It is characterized by muscular weakness, weight loss, and bone pain.

IV. Osteoporosis is the decrease in bone density or the increase in porosity of the bone, making it extremely fragile. The loss of bone mass makes bones so porous and weak that they become fragile and prone to fracture. Compression fractures of the vertebrae often occur as the result of osteoporosis and can lead to a decrease in height. The etiology of osteoporosis may be the aging process or a decrease in estrogen level that occurs after menopause.

V. Paget's disease, also known as *osteitis deformans,* is a condition of the adult skeleton in which localized areas of bone become hyperactive and overproduce. This hyperactive bone is replaced by a softer, enlarged osseous structure. The new bone is abnormal and tends to fracture easily.

VI. Fractures may result from excessive torque or stress on a bone. There are several types of fractures:
    A. *Simple or closed fracture:* a break in the bone that does not penetrate the skin (Fig. 5-1).
    B. *Compound or open fracture:* a break in the bone in which the skin is pierced or broken by the bone (Fig. 5-1).
    C. *Comminuted fracture:* a break in the bone in which the bone splinters or is crushed (Fig. 5-2).
    D. *Greenstick fracture:* a break in which the bone is cracked (i.e., broken on one side but bent on the other) (Fig. 5-3).
    E. *Pathological fracture:* a fracture that occurs spontaneously when bones are diseased (i.e., metastasized bone or bone affected by osteoporosis).
    F. *Compression fracture:* a fracture characterized by crushed bone[1] (Fig. 5-4).
    G. *Epiphyseal fracture:* a fracture at the growth plate of a long bone[1] (Fig. 5-5).
    H. *Avulsion fracture:* a fracture in which a piece of bone is pulled loose at the attachment of a tendon[1] (Fig. 5-6).
VII. Dislocations and sprains occur when a dislocated bone is forcibly separated from its joint.
    A. Dislocations most commonly occur in the shoulder due to the increased mobility and decreased stability of the joint. With dislocation ligaments and tendons are torn and must be immobilized to allow healing. Another common site of dislocation is the fingers (Fig. 5-7).
    B. Sprains occur when ligaments are twisted beyond their limits, leading to damage.
VIII. Neoplasia of bone refers to neoplasms or tumors of the bone that may be either malignant or benign. Such neoplasms may lead to fractures.
    A. *Osteoma:* the most common type of benign tumor of the bone. Osteomas may first appear as swelling and result in decreased range of motion of the involved joint. Surgical removal of the tumor may be required.

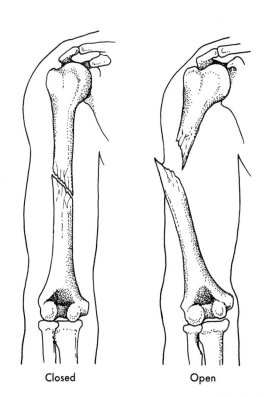

Closed   Open

FIG 5-1.   Open and closed fractures. (From Booher JM, Thibodeau GA: *Athletic injury assessment,* ed 3, St Louis, 1994, Mosby.)

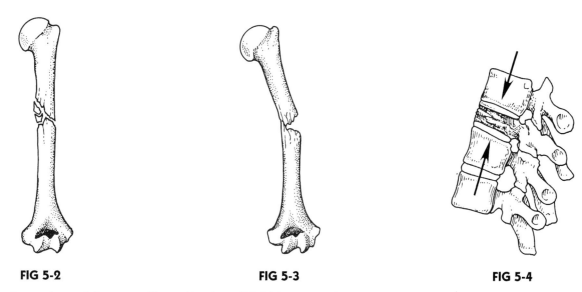

FIG 5-2   **FIG 5-3**   **FIG 5-4**

FIG 5-2.   Comminuted fracture. (From Booher JM, Thibodeau GA: *Athletic injury assessment,* ed 3, St Louis, 1994, Mosby.)

FIG 5-3.   Greenstick fracture. (From Booher JM, Thibodeau GA: *Athletic injury assessment,* ed 3, St Louis, 1994, Mosby.)

FIG 5-4.   Compression fracture. (From Booher JM, Thibodeau GA: *Athletic injury assessment,* ed 3, St Louis, 1994, Mosby.)

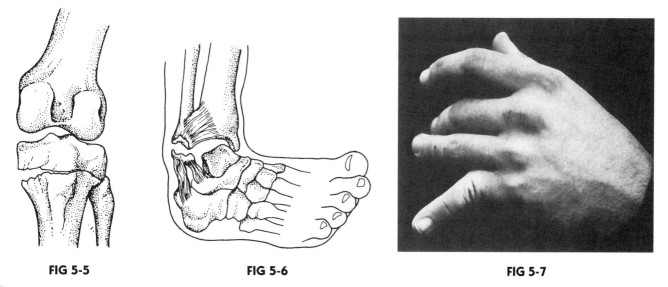

FIG 5-5   **FIG 5-6**   **FIG 5-7**

FIG 5-5.   Epiphyseal fracture. (From Booher JM, Thibodeau GA: *Athletic injury assessment,* ed 3, St Louis, 1994, Mosby.)

FIG 5-6.   Avulsion fracture. (From Booher JM, Thibodeau GA: *Athletic injury assessment,* ed 3, St Louis, 1994, Mosby.)

FIG 5-7.   Finger dislocation. (From Booher JM, Thibodeau GA: *Athletic injury assessment,* ed 3, St Louis, 1994, Mosby.)

B. *Giant cell tumors:* tumors that may be either benign or malignant. On x-ray films, these tumors appear as a collection of tubules. These tumors usually require surgical removal.

C. *Osteogenic sarcoma:* a primary malignancy of the bone that is usually located in the ends of long bones. It is most common in young people. The knee joint and tibia are the most frequently involved areas. Chemotherapy is usually given before the tumor removal to cause shrinkage of the tumor.

Diseases of the Joints

I. Arthritis is a disease characterized by inflammation of the joints. As you should remember from Chapter 1, *arthro-* means "joint" and *-itis* means "inflammation." The symptoms of arthritis are redness of joints, pain, swelling, and stiffness, especially in the morning.

A. Rheumatoid arthritis is the most disabling form of arthritis. It begins with inflammation of the synovial membrane. Rheumatoid arthritis affects young women more often than men. Its etiology is not known and there is no cure at this time. A juvenile type of rheumatoid arthritis also exists. Rheumatoid arthritis is characterized by periods of exacerbation and remission. It is considered a systemic disease, which means it can affect many different systems in the body. Diagnosis of rheumatoid arthritis is usually made by blood tests, such as the rheumatoid factor.

The effects of the disease can be diminished to some extent by early detection, an exercise program to maintain joint mobility, antiinflammatory medication to control the symptoms, and exercises to maintain good posture and minimize stress on the affected joints.

B. Osteoarthritis is the most common type of arthritis and is associated with aging. It is also referred to as "wear-and-tear" arthritis. Unlike rheumatoid arthritis, osteoarthritis may affect only one joint. Osteoarthritis begins in the articular cartilage rather than the synovial membrane. Diagnosis of osteoarthritis is usually made based on radiographic examination, patient history, and physical examination.

As with rheumatoid arthritis, there is no cure. The symptoms can be minimized with proper exercise, medication, and rest.

C. Gout is usually referred to as *gouty arthritis* and involves primarily the feet. The most common location in the foot is the large toe. This is a painful form of arthritis caused by uric acid deposits in the joints. Its etiology is unknown and is most common in middle-aged men. It is diagnosed by a blood test to determine the uric acid level in the blood.

Treatment involves medication to reduce the uric acid level and rest to decrease weight-bearing stress on the involved joints.

Diseases Affecting Specific Joints in the Body

I. Spine

A. Surface landmarks on the back

1. It is important to be familiar with these landmarks to understand how the bones and joints are affected by various diseases.

Surface landmarks	Spinal cord segment(s)
Vertebra prominens	C7
Top of scapula	T2
Base of spine of scapula	T4
Inferior angle of scapula	T7
Lowest rib insertion	T12
Top of iliac crest	L4
Dimples marking posterosuperior iliac spines	S1-S2

B. Cervical spine
  1. Segmental innervation and reflex testing
     a) Muscle strength in the upper extremities should be checked. Weakness in any of the following movements may be a sign of nerve impingement or disc involvement at the given level.

Movement	Spinal cord segment(s)
Neck flexion	C1
Neck rotation	C2
Neck lateral flexion	C3
Shoulder shrug	C4
Shoulder abduction	C5
Elbow flexion	C6
Wrist extension	C6
Elbow extension	C7
Wrist flexion	C7-8
Thumb extension	C8
Finger abduction	C8, T1

  b) Upper limb reflexes should be checked when there is a sensory (dermatome) deficit.[1] Figs. 5-8 and 5-9 give examples of reflex tests for C5-8.

Muscle	Spinal cord segment(s)
Biceps brachii	C5-6 (Fig. 5-8)
Brachioradialis	C6 (Fig. 5-9)
Triceps brachii	C7, C8 (Fig. 5-8)

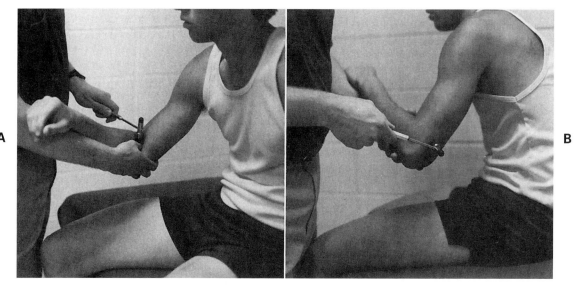

A   B

FIG 5-8. **A,** Biceps reflex. **B,** Triceps reflex. (From Booher JM, Thibodeau GA: *Athletic injury assessment,* ed 3, St Louis, 1994, Mosby.)

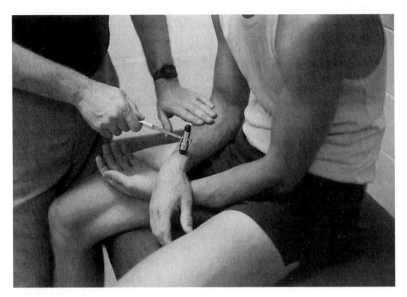

FIG 5-9. Brachioradialis reflex. (From Booher JM, Thibodeau GA: *Athletic injury assessment,* ed 3, St Louis, 1994, Mosby.)

    2. Disorders

      a) Brachial plexus neuritis is characterized by intense shoulder pain. Usually there is no history of injury, but this pain may occur after strenuous activity and may be accompanied by muscle weakness. Treatment involves two phases: (1) initial rest of the involved area until the pain decreases followed by (2) rehabilitation and strengthening of the involved muscles.

      b) Acute torticollis is also called *wryneck.* The head assumes a cocked position (laterally flexed and rotated)[2] (Fig. 5-10).

      c) Whiplash is also called *acceleration injury.* The mechanism of the injury is usually a car accident in which a car is struck from behind. The individual's torso is usually thrown forward, whereas the neck is thrust backward into hyperextension (Fig. 5-11).

      d) Acute disc bulge occurs when the nucleus pulposus pushes or tears a weakened anulus. If the disc bulges anteriorly, it presses on the anterior longitudinal ligament and may cause spasm of the longus colli muscle. If the disc bulges posteriorly, it may press on the posterior longitudinal ligament, spinal cord, or nerve root.

  C. Lumbosacral spine

    1. Segmental innervation and reflex testing

Movement	Spinal cord segment(s)
Hip flexion	L2-3
Knee extension	L3-4
Foot dorsiflexion	L4-5
Extension of large toe	L5
Ankle eversion	S1
Hip extension	L5-S1
Knee flexion	L5-S1

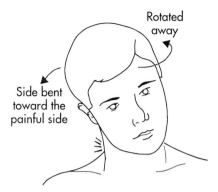

FIG 5-10. Acute torticollis (wryneck). (From Hartley A: *Practical joint assessment: upper quadrant,* ed 2, St Louis, 1995, Mosby.)

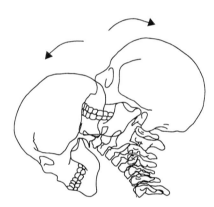

FIG 5-11. Whiplash mechanism. (From Hartley A: *Practical joint assessment: upper quadrant,* ed 2, St Louis, 1995, Mosby.)

2. Disorders
   a) Spondylolysis is a defect in the neural arch, usually in the pars interarticularis.
   b) Spondylolisthesis is a slipping of one vertebra forward over another.
   c) Ankylosing spondylitis (Marie-Strümpell disease) is an inflammatory disorder that affects the spine.
   d) Scheuermann's disease is an inflammatory disorder in which changes occur in the end-plate of the vertebra, especially the anterior body. It is more common in girls than boys.
   e) Reiter's syndrome is a condition comprised of urethritis, conjunctivitis, and some form of arthritis. It is a disease of young people and is thought to be a venereal-type disease.
   f) Scoliosis is a deformity in which there are one or more lateral curvatures of the lumbar or thoracic spine. There are two types:
      (1) *Functional:* caused by poor posture, hysteria, nerve root irritation, leg-length discrepancy, unilateral muscle imbalance, or unilateral muscle tightness.
      (2) *Structural:* may be caused by any of the following: hereditary growth abnormality, structural leg-length discrepancy, or structural pelvis obliquity.

II. Shoulder

    A. Impingement syndrome involves the pinching of the supraspinatus and/or biceps tendon in the coracoacromial arch, usually during abduction. Impingement syndrome can produce progressive degenerative changes in the affected structures. It often begins as tendinitis, especially in the supraspinatus or biceps tendon. Tendinitis causes edema and hemorrhage, leading to stage 1 impingement. In stage 2, thickening and fibrosis of the soft tissue occur. Stage 3 involves rotator cuff tears, bicep tendon ruptures, and skeletal changes[2] (Fig. 5-12).

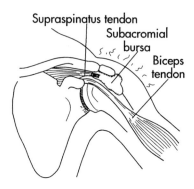

Supraspinatus tendon
Subacromial bursa
Biceps tendon

FIG 5-12. Subacromial impingement. (From Hartley A: *Practical joint assessment: upper quadrant,* ed 2, St Louis, 1995, Mosby.)

    B. Acromioclavicular joint separation can be described in three degrees according to severity.

        1. First-degree separation is a mild sprain, which leads to stretching and an incomplete tear of the acromioclavicular ligament. Tenderness directly over the joint and minimal swelling occur. No disability to the shoulder results.

        2. Second-degree separation is a complete tear of the acromioclavicular ligament and incomplete tear of the coracoclavicular ligament. Tenderness directly over the joint, swelling, and increased pain with forced range of motion occurs. These symptoms may or may not be accompanied by upward displacement of the clavicle.

        3. Third-degree separation is a complete tear of the acromioclavicular and coracoclavicular ligaments. The patient exhibits differing degrees of tenderness, swelling, joint instability, and increased pain with any amount of range of motion. There is severe upward riding of the clavicle. The acromioclavicular joint exhibits the *piano key sign.* This sign occurs when the clavicle springs back up after pressure is applied to the clavicle and then released.[2]

    C. Adhesive capsulitis (frozen shoulder) is a condition characterized by capsular thickening, contraction, adhesions, and decreased synovial fluid. The greatest restrictions in decreasing order are external rotation, abduction, forward flexion, and internal rotation.

    D. Rotator cuff tear occurs when one of the muscles or tendons forming the rotator cuff is lacerated. The most common tendon involved is the supraspinatus tendon and the most common weakness is in external rotation.

    E. Shoulder dislocation can be labeled as anterior, posterior, or multidirectional.

        1. *Anterior:* common throwing injury. Deltoid muscle atrophy or anterior glenoid damage may be present. The arm is held in slight abduction (approximately 15 to 20 degrees). It is important to strengthen the infraspinatus muscle due to its function in pulling the humeral head posteriorly.

2. *Posterior:* usually the result of a stretched posterior capsule. It can also occur with the fracture of posterior glenoid, stretched subscapularis tendon, and avulsion of the subscapularis tendon and lesser tuberosity. The arm is held in adduction and internal rotation.

3. *Multidirectional:* combination of anterior and posterior dislocation.

F. Thoracic outlet syndrome consists of a group of syndromes resulting from compression of the thoracic neurovascular bundle, which includes the brachial plexus, subclavian artery, and subclavian vein. This neurovascular bundle runs from the thorax through an outlet formed by the scalene muscles and the first rib.[2] Some of the symptoms are drooping shoulder girdle, continual hyperabduction of the arm, numbness, cyanosis, and edema of affected arm.

III. Elbow

A. Tennis elbow (lateral epicondylitis) affects the tendinous origin of the wrist extensors and supinator muscles. It can be caused by faulty techniques in racket sports, weak or poorly conditioned muscles, or poorly fitted equipment (Fig. 5-13).

B. Golfer's elbow (medial epicondylitis or "little league elbow") affects the common flexor origin. It is tested for with Tinel's sign, which involves tapping the ulnar nerve (Fig. 5-14).

C. Posterior elbow dislocation is the posterior displacement of the ulna (olecranon is shifted backward and upward) in relationship to the humerus. As the elbow is forced into hyperextension, the collateral ligaments are stretched or ruptured, allowing the posterior shifting of the ulna (Fig. 5-15). This injury is not common.

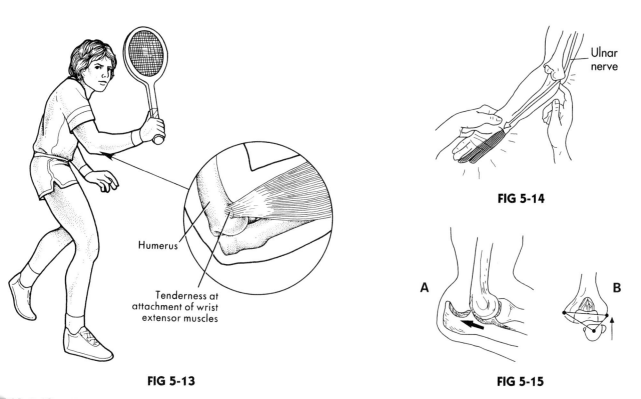

FIG 5-13

Humerus

Tenderness at attachment of wrist extensor muscles

Ulnar nerve

FIG 5-14

A   B

FIG 5-15

FIG 5-13.   Tennis elbow (lateral epicondylitis). (From Booher JM, Thibodeau GA: *Athletic injury assessment,* ed 3, St Louis, 1994, Mosby.)

FIG 5-14.   Golfer's elbow (medial epicondylitis). (From Hartley A: *Practical joint assessment: upper quadrant,* ed 2, St Louis, 1995, Mosby.)

FIG 5-15.   **A,** Posterior elbow dislocation. **B,** Posterior view of bony alignment. (From Hartley A: *Practical joint assessment: upper quadrant,* ed 2, St Louis, 1995, Mosby.)

IV. Wrist and finger

A. Carpal tunnel syndrome (median nerve entrapment) is usually thought of as an overuse syndrome associated with flexor tendinitis on the palmar surface of the wrist. The patient may have sensory loss in the median nerve distribution (Fig. 5-16).

1. *Phalen's test:* forced wrist flexion, which if positive causes tingling or numbness in the thumb, index, or middle finger within 60 seconds (Fig. 5-17).

2. *Tinel's sign:* median nerve percussion test. Tapping over the center of the carpal tunnel at the wrist may produce tingling or paresthesia distal to the point of pressure (see Fig. 5-14).

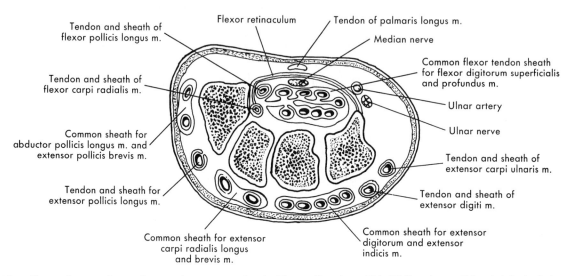

FIG 5-16. Carpal tunnel syndrome (cross section). (From Booher JM, Thibodeau GA: *Athletic injury assessment,* ed 3, St Louis, 1994, Mosby.)

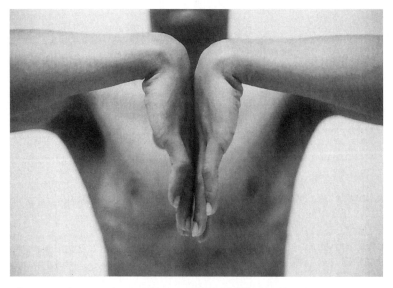

FIG 5-17. Phalen's test for carpal tunnel syndrome. (From Booher JM, Thibodeau GA: *Athletic injury assessment,* ed 3, St Louis, 1994, Mosby.)

  B. Reflex sympathetic dystrophy is a vasomotor disorder characterized by hyperesthesia, burning pain, edema, discoloration, and stiffness.

  C. Colles' fracture involves a dorsally angulated and displaced distal radial fracture that may also include an additional avulsion or fracture of the tip of the ulnar styloid process (Fig. 5-18).

  D. Raynaud's phenomenon includes painful vasoconstriction followed by vasodilation. The vasoconstriction is most often triggered by cold.

  E. De Quervain's tenosynovitis is the most common form of tendonitis in the wrist. It involves inflammation of the tendons of the first dorsal compartment of the wrist (i.e., abductor pollicis longus and extensor pollicis brevis). It is diagnosed by the Finkelstein test (Fig. 5-19). The patient makes a fist with the thumb flexed inside the hand. The patient then ulnar deviates his/her wrist. If pain occurs with this movement, the test is positive.

  F. Mallet finger is a common injury and is usually the result of forced flexion of the distal phalanx while the extensor tendons are actively trying to extend the digit (Fig. 5-20).

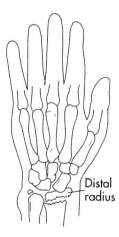

FIG 5-18. Colles' fracture. (From Hartley A: *Practical joint assessment: upper quadrant,* ed 2, St Louis, 1995, Mosby.)

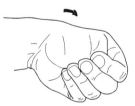

FIG 5-19. Finkelstein test for de Quervain's syndrome. (From Hartley A: *Practical joint assessment: upper quadrant,* ed 2, St Louis, 1995, Mosby.)

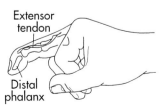

FIG 5-20. Mallet finger. (From Hartley A: *Practical joint assessment: upper quadrant,* ed 2, St Louis, 1995, Mosby.)

V. Hip, pelvis and sacroiliac joint
    A. Bursitis of the hip afflicts three major sites (Fig. 5-21): (1) greater trochanteric bursa, (2) ischial bursa, and (3) psoas bursa.
    B. Osteoarthritis (degenerative joint disease) is the most common disorder of the hip joint. It is also referred to as "wear-and-tear" arthritis. The afflicted person is usually middle aged and complains of sudden-onset pain near the groin or trochanteric area.
    C. Acetabular fractures are usually the result of the femoral head being driven forcefully into the acetabulum.
    D. Hip dislocations occur when an external force causes the hip to dislocate. Because of the structural stability of the hip joint, the external force required to dislocate the hip is severe. The hip may dislocate in two directions.
        1. Posterior dislocation results from a force that causes a combination of flexion, adduction, and internal rotation (Fig. 5-22).
        2. Anterior dislocation results from a force that causes a combination of slight flexion, abduction, and external rotation.
    E. Hip pointer is caused by a severe blow to the unprotected iliac crest (e.g., a blow to the iliac crest with an opponent's football helmet).
    F. Piriformis syndrome is the entrapment of the sciatic nerve at the point where it emerges from the pelvis through the greater sciatic foramen, passing between the piriformis muscle above and the obturator internus muscle below.
    G. Avascular necrosis of the hip is the avascular necrosis of the head of the femur. It may follow trauma or occur as a complication of another disease. The arterial blood supply is interrupted, which may be the result of a fracture of the femoral neck, slipped femoral epiphysis, dislocation of the hip, or fall on the hip.
    H. Coxa vara (genu valgum) is a deformity of the hip in which the angle formed by the axis of the head and neck of the femur and the axis of the shaft of the femur (called the *angle of inclination of the hip*) is less than 125 degrees (Fig. 5-23). The normal angle is 125 degrees.
    I. Coxa valga (genu varum) of the hip is a deformity of the hip in which the angle formed by the axis of the head and neck of the femur and the axis of the shaft of the femur is greater than 125 degrees (Fig. 5-23).

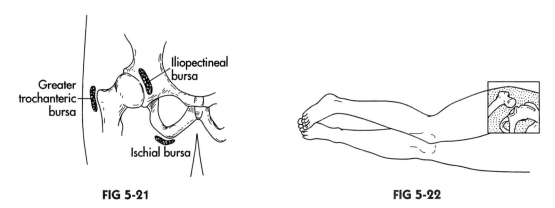

FIG 5-21

FIG 5-22

FIG 5-21. Hip bursae locations. (From Hartley A: *Practical joint assessment: lower quadrant,* ed 2, St Louis, 1995, Mosby.)

FIG 5-22. Posterior hip dislocation. (From Hartley A: *Practical joint assessment: lower quadrant,* ed 2, St Louis, 1995, Mosby.)

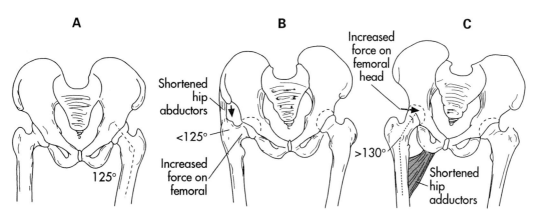

FIG 5-23. **A,** Normal anterior view. **B,** Coxa vara. **C,** Coxa valga. (From Hartley A: *Practical joint assessment: lower quadrant,* ed 2, St Louis, 1995, Mosby.)

VI. Knee
    A. Ligamentous instability
        1. Anterior instability is identified if the tibia is displaced anteriorly in relationship to the femur (anterior drawer sign) (Fig. 5-24). This test is performed with the patient lying supine with the knee flexed to 90 degrees. The foot is stabilized by the examiner sitting on the forefoot. The examiner pulls forward on the proximal part of the calf.
        2. Posterior instability is identified if the tibia is displaced posteriorly in relationship to the femur (posterior drawer sign) (Fig. 5-25). This test is performed with the patient lying supine with the knee flexed to 90 degrees. The foot is stabilized by the examiner sitting on the forefoot. The examiner grasps the calf and attempts to move the tibia backward.
        3. Medial instability is identified by a positive abduction or valgus test (Fig. 5-26). This test is performed by applying a valgus or lateral force with the patient's knee in about 20 degrees of flexion and externally rotated slightly. Excessive movement of the tibia away from the femur indicates damage to the medial collateral ligament.
        4. Lateral instability is identified by a positive adduction or varus test (Fig. 5-27). This test is performed by applying a varus or medial force with the patient's knee in about 20 degrees of flexion. Excessive movement of the tibia away from the femur indicates damage to the lateral collateral ligament.

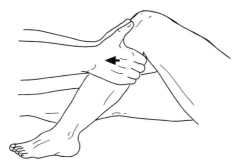

FIG 5-24. Anterior drawer test. (From Hartley A: *Practical joint assessment: lower quadrant,* ed 2, St Louis, 1995, Mosby.)

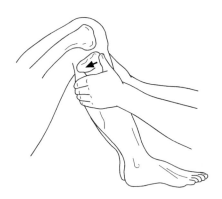

FIG 5-25. Posterior drawer test. (From Hartley A: *Practical joint assessment: lower quadrant,* ed 2, St Louis, 1995, Mosby.)

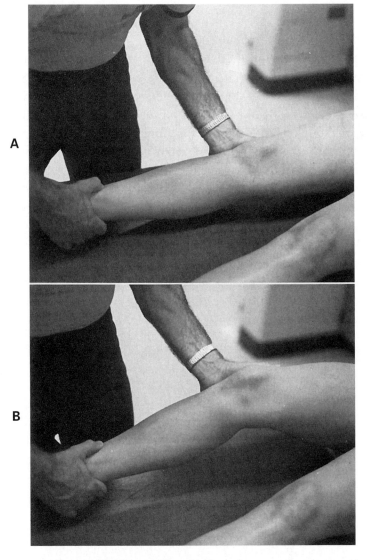

FIG 5-26. Abduction stress test for medial instability. **A,** Knee in complete extension. **B,** Knee at approximately 30 degrees of flexion. (From Booher JM, Thibodeau GA: *Athletic injury assessment,* ed 3, St Louis, 1994, Mosby.)

B. Patellar tendinitis (jumper's knee) occurs as an overuse syndrome in many active athletes (e.g., runners, dancers, jumpers). The quadriceps femoris muscle becomes the patellar tendon at its distal attachment, which runs from the lower part of the patella to its insertion on the tibial tubercle.

C. Osgood-Schlatter disease is a type of osteochondritis associated with the partial tear or avulsion of the patellar tendon at its insertion at the tibial tubercle. Many times an enlargement of the tibial tubercle can be seen on x-ray film (Fig. 5-28).

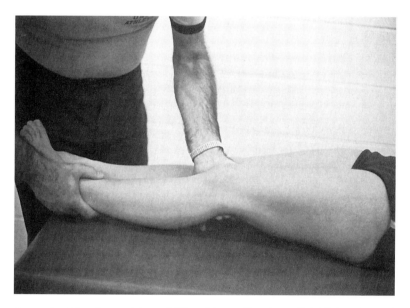

FIG 5-27. Adduction stress test for lateral instability. (From Booher JM, Thibodeau GA: *Athletic injury assessment,* ed 3, St Louis, 1994, Mosby.)

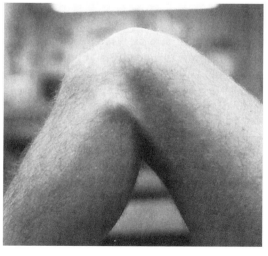

FIG 5-28. Osgood-Schlatter disease. (From Booher JM, Thibodeau GA: *Athletic injury assessment,* ed 3, St Louis, 1994, Mosby.)

D. Chondromalacia of the patella is a common disorder of the articular cartilage of the patella. The lesions in the cartilage are due to premature degeneration, with softening and roughening of the cartilage. Many times individuals with this disorder have weak vastus medialis obliquus muscle.

E. Iliotibial band syndrome is an overuse injury caused by friction in the bursa, which is over the laterofemoral condyle, and the iliotibial band. The patient complains of pain on the lateral side of the knee where the iliotibial band passes over the laterofemoral condyle when the knee is extended slowly from the 90-degree flexed position. The greatest pain is produced at the 30-degree flexed position.

VII. Ankle and calf

A. Achilles tendon rupture may be a complete or partial rupture. The location of the rupture is usually approximately 5 cm above the tendon insertion (Fig. 5-29). The usual symptoms are:

1. Visible defect in the tendon
2. Inability to perform heel raises on one leg
3. Swelling and discoloration around the malleoli
4. Failure of the foot to plantar flex when the examiner squeezes the gastrocnemius (Thompson test)
5. Excessive passive dorsiflexion

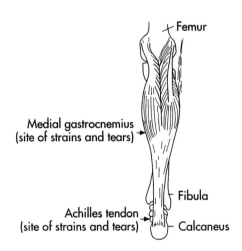

FIG 5-29.   Achilles tendon injury sites. (From Hartley A: *Practical joint assessment: lower quadrant,* ed 2, St Louis, 1995, Mosby.)

B. Lateral collateral ligament sprain most often occurs by excessive inversion that occurs at the same time as plantar flexion (Fig. 5-30). The lateral collateral ligament is comprised of anterior fibers (anterior talofibular ligament), medial fibers (fibulocalcaneal ligament), and posterior fibers (posterior talofibular ligament).

C. Medial ligament sprains are not as common as lateral collateral ligament sprains due to the size of the medial ligament (deltoid ligament). They are primarily caused by forced eversion and plantar flexion.

D. Tarsal tunnel syndrome is a compression syndrome that involves the tibial nerve.

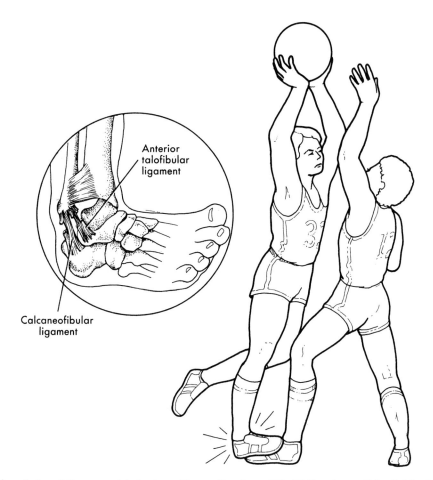

FIG 5-30. Lateral collateral ligament injuries. (From Booher JM, Thibodeau GA: *Athletic injury assessment,* ed 3, St Louis, 1994, Mosby.)

NEUROLOGICAL DISORDERS

The body has only one nervous system, even though we sometimes think of some of its subdivisions as individual systems. As discussed in Chapter 4, the subdivisions of the nervous system are the central nervous system (CNS) and the peripheral nervous system (PNS).

Disorders of the Central Nervous System

I. Infectious diseases
   A. Meningitis is an inflammation of the meninges of the brain or spinal cord. It usually involves the first two meninges of the brain or spinal cord (pia mater and arachnoid). It can be caused by a bacteria or a virus and usually affects children more often than adults. The symptoms of meningitis are headaches, high fever, chills, and stiff neck. Diagnosis of meningitis is made by the use of lumbar punctures.
   B. Encephalitis is an inflammation of the brain and meninges caused most often by a viral infection. Some think that the virus is carried by wild birds and transmitted to humans by mosquitoes. Symptoms are headaches, fever, paralysis, coma, and seizures. Diagnosis of encephalitis is made by use of lumbar punctures.

   C. Poliomyelitis is an infection of the brain and spinal cord caused by a virus. This disease is extremely rare since the development of the Salk and Sabin vaccines and immunization programs. The areas of prime involvement are the motor neurons of the spinal cord and medulla oblongata. Symptoms are headaches, fever, sore throat, and stomach disorders.

 II. Degenerative neural disorders

   A. Multiple sclerosis is a gradually progressing CNS disorder. It is characterized by disseminated areas of demyelination of the brain and spinal cord. The demyelination results in many varied symptoms such as muscle weakness; poor balance and coordination; and paresthesia in one or more extremities, trunk, and face. It is difficult to diagnose and has periods of remissions and exacerbations. It affects young adults between 20 and 40 years of age. There is no successful treatment for multiple sclerosis.

   B. Parkinson's disease is a gradually progressing degenerative disease of the CNS. It is also known as "pill roller's disease" or "shaking palsy." Symptoms include a pill roller's tremor of the hand, nodding of the head, slowness of movement, muscle rigidity, and postural instability. Most of the degeneration of nerve cells occurs in the basal ganglia (area controlling body movements). Treatment includes the use of levadopa, which is converted to dopamine (neural transmitter substance) in the brain. The cause of Parkinson's disease is unknown.

   C. Huntington's chorea is an inherited disease with symptoms that may not appear until middle age. A major symptom is loss of muscle control. Other symptoms include personality changes, poor judgment, impaired memory, dementia, and physical symptoms such as jerking, twisting, and muscle spasm. The disease is fast progressing and has no known treatment.

   D. Cerebrovascular accident is a condition also referred to as a *stroke.* It is caused by an embolism, thrombosis, hemorrhage, or vasospasm of the cerebral blood vessels. This event leads to an infarct (cell death) due to a lack of blood supply to the brain. Symptoms vary depending on the location of the infarct. The symptoms by location of the cerebrovascular accident are:

     1. Left hemisphere of the brain

       a) Muscle weakness or paralysis on the right side of the body

       b) Aphasia

       c) Decreased ability to discriminate between right and left

       d) Right hemianopia

     2. Right hemisphere of the brain

       a) Muscle weakness or paralysis on the left side of the body

       b) Decreased attention span and judgment

       c) Diminished ability to perform abstract reasoning

       d) Left hemianopia

       e) Emotional instability

       f) Reduced spatial orientation

       g) Memory loss

     3. Cerebellum

       a) Lack of postural righting ability

       b) Lack of balance and coordination

       c) Ataxia

       d) Nystagmus

     4. Brainstem

       a) Decreased muscle strength on both sides

       b) Paralysis on both sides

       c) Fluctuating vital signs

       d) Difficulty swallowing

III. Spinal cord injuries
   A. Spinal cord injuries by level of injury

Level of injury	Muscles innervated	Available movements
C1-3	Face, neck	Talking, sipping, blowing
C4	Diaphragm	Respiration (40% to 50%)
	Trapezius	Scapular elevation
C5	Deltoid	Shoulder flexion, abduction
	Biceps brachii	Elbow flexion
	Rhomboid major and rhomboid minor	Scapular adduction
	External rotators	Shoulder external rotation
C6	Extensor carpi radialis	Wrist extension
	Infraspinatus	Shoulder external rotation
	Latissimus dorsi (weak)	Shoulder extension and external rotation
	Serratus anterior	Scapular abduction
	Pronator teres	Forearm pronation
	Pectoralis major (clavicular)	Shoulder external rotation
C7	Extensor pollicis longus and extensor pollicis brevis	Finger extension
	Triceps brachii	Elbow extension
	Flexor carpi radialis	Wrist flexion
C8-T1	Finger extensors	Full innervation of upper extremity muscles
	Flexor carpi ulnaris	
	Flexor pollicis longus and flexor pollicis brevis	
	Lumbricales, opponens	
T4-6	Top one half of intercostals	Improved trunk control
	Long muscles of back	Increased respiratory capacity
T9-12	All intercostals	Increased endurance
	Lower abdominals	Full trunk control
L1-3	Pectineus, gracilis	Hip flexion and adduction
	Iliopsoas	Hip flexion
	Rectus femoris	Hip flexion, knee extension
	Sartorius	Hip flexion, abduction, external rotation
L4-5	Quadriceps femoris	Hip flexion, knee extension
	Hamstrings (short head) (L5-S1)	Hip extension, knee flexion
	Lower erector spinae	Back extension
	Tibialis anterior	Dorsiflexion, inversion
	Tibialis posterior	Plantar flexion, inversion of foot

Disorders of the Peripheral Nervous System

I. Injuries to the brachial plexus
   A. Upper brachial plexus injury (Erb-Duchenne paralysis) is the most prevalent of all brachial plexus injuries and is caused by damage to the roots of C5 and C6. It occurs with traction or compression injuries.
   B. Lower brachial plexus injury (Klumpke's paralysis) occurs when there is damage to the roots of C8 and T1. This disorder is caused by birth injury.

C. Specific peripheral nerve injuries

Nerve	Symptoms
Long thoracic	Winging of scapula (weakness of serratus anterior) (Fig. 5-31)
Anterior thoracic	Paralysis or weakness of pectoralis major and pectoralis minor muscles
Dorsal scapular	Paralysis or weakness of the rhomboid muscles
Suprascapular	Weakness of supraspinatus and infraspinatus muscles
Axillary	Paralysis of the deltoid muscle with loss of contour of the shoulder and difficulty flexing, abducting, and extending shoulder
Musculocutaneous	Paralysis of the biceps brachii and brachialis muscles leading to weakness in elbow flexion and supination
Median	Paralysis of the thenar muscles leading to the loss of opposition (ape hand deformity) (Fig. 5-32)
Ulnar	Results in the claw hand deformity; loss of use of the interossei muscles (no abduction or adduction); inability to flex the proximal or distal phalanges of the fourth or fifth digits; first phalanges of these fingers are hyperextended; fifth finger is abducted (Fig. 5-33)
Radial	Results in inability to extend the wrist fingers or thumb (sometimes referred to as *wrist drop*) (Fig. 5-34)

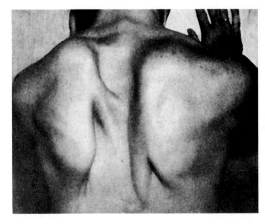

FIG 5-31.   Winging of left scapula due to injury of the long thoracic nerve. (From Booher JM, Thibodeau GA: *Athletic injury assessment,* ed 3, St Louis, 1994, Mosby.)

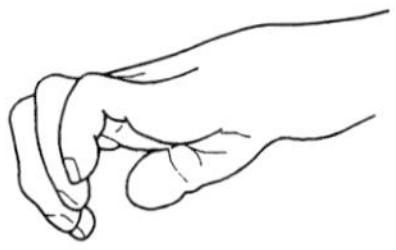

FIG 5-32 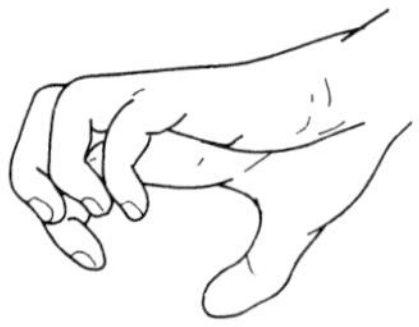   **FIG 5-33** 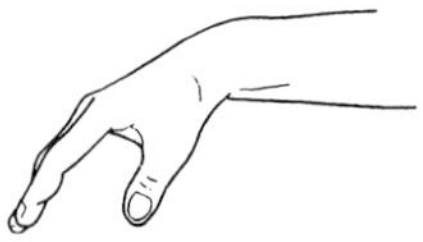   **FIG 5-34**

FIG 5-32.   Median nerve injury: "ape hand." (From Hartley A: *Practical joint assessment: upper quadrant,* ed 2, St Louis, 1995, Mosby.)

FIG 5-33.   Ulnar nerve injury: "claw hand." (From Hartley A: *Practical joint assessment: upper quadrant,* ed 2, St Louis, 1995, Mosby.)

FIG 5-34.   Radial nerve injury: "wrist drop." (From Hartley A: *Practical joint assessment: upper quadrant,* ed 2, St Louis, 1995, Mosby.)

II. Injuries to the lumbar plexus
  A. Injuries to the lumbar plexus are rare because the lumbar plexus lies deep within the abdomen in the psoas major muscle.
  B. Specific peripheral nerve injuries

Nerve	Symptoms
Ilioinguinal	Of little significance; possible pain when standing
Obturator	Weakness of adduction and internal and external rotation of thigh; nerve can be damaged during labor or delivery
Femoral	Paralysis of the iliopsoas muscle, which causes an inability to flex the thigh to the chest

III. Injuries to the sacral plexus
  A. Injuries to the sacral plexus are rare but can occur with disc disease, fractures, or dislocations.
  B. Specific peripheral nerve injuries

Nerve	Symptoms
Sciatic	Loss of knee flexion; foot drop is very prevalent
Tibial	Loss of plantar flexion, adduction, inversion
Common peroneal	Paralysis of the muscles of the anterior and lateral compartments of the calf; foot drop is common
Deep peroneal	Loss of dorsiflexion
Superficial peroneal	Inability to evert the foot

PULMONARY DISORDERS

The respiratory system moves air into and out of the lungs. This system moves the gases in the air into the body so that tissues and blood can use them. Several disorders interfere with this process.
  I. Chronic obstructive pulmonary disease (COPD) is a disease that increases the resistance to air passing into and out of the lungs. It is characterized by slowed expiration, which is thought to be caused by a narrowing of the bronchial tubes. It includes asthma, bronchitis, bronchiectasis, and emphysema.
    A. Asthma is a pulmonary disease characterized by:
      1. Airway obstruction that is reversible either spontaneously or with treatment
      2. Airway inflammation
      3. Predisposition for hypersensitivity to various allergens
      4. Wheezing and difficulty breathing
    B. Bronchitis is acute inflammation of the bronchial tree. Symptoms consist of chilling, slight fever, back and muscle spasm or pain, coughing, wheezing, and sore throat.
    C. Bronchiectasis usually exists due to an already existing disease. The suffix -ectasis means "dilation." Bronchiectasis is an irreversible, bronchial dilation caused by infection. Many times it is associated with a congenital or hereditary condition or can be a complication of influenza, pneumonia, or a chronic sinus infection.
    D. Emphysema is a chronic obstructive pulmonary disease that is neither contagious nor infectious. The word emphysema means "inflation." The lungs become filled with stale air that is high in carbon dioxide content. The air cannot be completely exhaled to allow oxygen to refill the lungs. Most patients complain of a suffocating feeling and have an increased rate of breathing. Their appearance is characterized by a "barrel chest." The difficulty in breathing results from a loss of the elasticity of the lung tissue.
  II. Pneumothorax occurs when air gets in the pleural cavity between the visceral and pleural spaces. If air enters the pleural cavity, the lung collapses.
  III. Atelectasis occurs when air enters the pleural cavity and causes the collapse of the lungs.

BURNS

Burns can be caused by various sources such as contact with (1) fire directly, (2) hot surfaces, (3) boiling liquids, (4) chemicals, and (5) electricity.

To understand burns, a brief review of the structure of normal skin is needed. The skin is divided into three layers: (1) epidermis, (2) dermis, and (3) subcutaneous layer.

    I. The *epidermis,* or outer layer, has little vascular supply but controls body fluid and heat as well as provides skin color. This layer regenerates quickly.

    II. The *dermis,* the next layer, is much different in structure and function from the epidermis. Nerves, blood vessels, lymph glands, and sweat glands are located in the dermis.

    III. The *subcutaneous layer,* the third layer, is directly above the muscles, tendons, ligaments, and organs.

Depth of Burns

The depth of a burn may be classified according to its appearance and by the damage it causes to the various layers of skin. The classes are (1) first degree, (2) second degree, and (3) third degree.

    I. *First-degree burns* are red (like sunburns), sensitive to the touch, and moist. There are no blisters and they usually heal in 1 week or less.

    II. *Second-degree (superficial-thickness) burns* may or may not have blisters. This burn results in damage to the epidermis and possibly to the superficial part of the dermis. It is painful and may result in permanent skin color changes. It heals independently within 8 to 10 days.

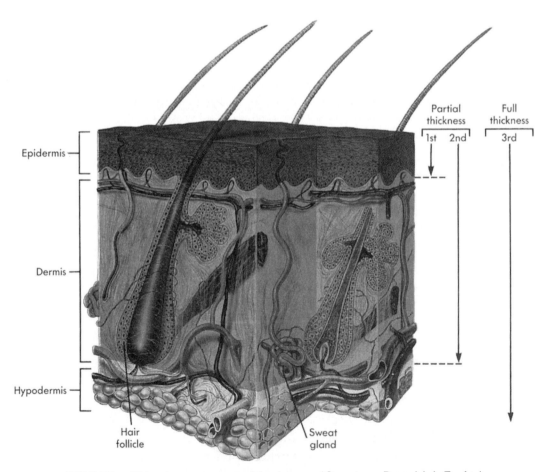

FIG 5-35. Skin damage caused by burns. (Courtesy Ronald J. Ervin.)

III. *Second-degree (deep) burns* cause damage to the entire epidermis as well as to much of the dermis. Many of the sweat glands and hair follicles are destroyed. More bleeding occurs with this burn than with first-degree burns because of the number of vessels in the dermis. The burn is painful because not all of the nerve endings are destroyed. The burn heals independently in 20 to 30 days.

IV. *Third-degree burns* destroy the entire epidermis and dermis. These burns do not heal on their own and cause severe edema and necrosis of the tissue. Usually there is no pain because the nerve endings are destroyed. Skin grafting is required for healing (Fig. 5-35).

Types of Grafts

I. An *allograft or homograft* is skin taken from another person. Often cadaver skin is used. The skin can be kept in a skin bank for extended periods of time. Allografts are temporary grafts used to cover large burns when there is not enough of the individual's own skin available for grafts.

II. An *autograft* is skin taken from a part of the burn victim's own body and used in another part of the body to cover a burn site. Common donor sites are the thighs, buttocks, and trunk. Autografts are the most preferred graft because the reinfection rate is much lower and they are permanent, therefore increasing the speed of healing.

III. A *heterograft or xenograft* is a graft of skin taken from another species. The heterografts used most often for humans are grafts taken from pigs. These grafts are temporary and again are used when large areas of burned tissue exist.

IV. A *full-thickness graft* consists of all layers of skin but no subcutaneous fat.

V. A *split-thickness graft* consists of superficial dermis only.

Rule of Nines

The rule of nines is a method used to estimate the percentage of body surface damaged by a burn. This system divides the body into areas that are approximately 9% or multiples of 9% (i.e., 4.5%, 18%) of the total body surface: head and neck (front and back); anterior trunk; posterior trunk and buttocks; genitalia and perineum; and anterior and posterior surfaces of the left arm, right arm, left leg, and right leg (Fig. 5-36).

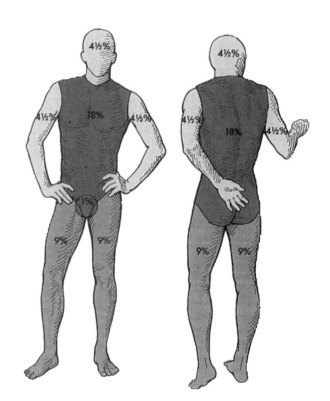

FIG 5-36. Rule of nines. (Courtesy G. David Brown.)

REVIEW QUESTIONS

1. A 21-year-old man is sent to your clinic for treatment. His chief complaint is pain over the medial epicondyle of the left elbow. This condition is most likely which of the following?
   a. Golfer's elbow
   b. Tennis elbow
   c. Softball elbow
   d. Biceps elbow

2. You are seeing a patient who states that her physician told her that she has a progressive contracture of the palmar fascia. She has a flexion contracture of the ring finger. What medical term would you use to describe her condition?
   a. Dupuytren's contracture
   b. Trigger finger
   c. Mallet finger
   d. Gamekeeper's finger

3. A 48-year-old man complains of low back pain. X-ray film shows that the L4 vertebra is slipping forward on the L5 vertebra. What term is used for this condition?
   a. Stenosis
   b. Scoliosis
   c. Spondylolisthesis
   d. Spondylosis

4. You see a newborn who has been diagnosed as having Klumpke's paralysis. What spinal level is injured?
   a. L1-2
   b. T2-4
   c. C8-T1
   d. C5-7

5. You are working with a patient who has experienced cerebrovascular accident (CVA). He is showing behavior of high anxiety, is quick to get angry, and is easily frustrated. What type of CVA do you think this patient has suffered?
   a. Right hemisphere
   b. Left hemisphere
   c. Frontal lobe
   d. None of the above

6. A burn patient has burns on the left anterior and posterior arm and anterior trunk. According to the rule of nines, what percentage of her body is burned?
   a. 18%
   b. 9%
   c. 27%
   d. 32%

7. The chief muscle responsible for respiration is the diaphragm. Which nerve innervates the diaphragm?
   a. Vagus
   b. Phrenic
   c. Hypoglossal
   d. Long thoracic

8. You are assisting a CVA patient with walking. She has muscle weakness on her right side, has aphasia, and cannot tell her right from her left side. Which area of the brain would you expect to be affected?
   a. Cerebellum
   b. Frontal lobe
   c. Right hemisphere
   d. Left hemisphere
9. A disease of early childhood in which a vitamin D deficiency does not allow the bones to properly ossify is:
   a. Pott's disease
   b. Osteomalacia
   c. Rickets
   d. Paget's disease
10. Paget's disease is also known as:
    a. Osteochondritis
    b. Osteomalacia
    c. Osteitis deformans
    d. None of the above
11. Pott's disease is a form of:
    a. Tuberculosis
    b. Osteoarthritis
    c. COPD
    d. Sarcoma
12. A fracture that occurs spontaneously when bones are diseased is:
    a. Greenstick
    b. Pathological
    c. Comminuted
    d. Compound
13. Rheumatoid arthritis begins with inflammation of the:
    a. Cartilage
    b. Bone
    c. Synovial membrane
    d. None of the above
14. The base of the spine of the scapula is a surface landmark for what vertebral level?
    a. T7
    b. T10
    c. T4
    d. C8
15. The vertebra prominens is found at what level?
    a. C3
    b. C6
    c. C7
    d. L1

16. A 64-year-old man tells you he smokes a minimum of one pack of cigarettes a day, he has a barrel-shaped chest, and he complains of being short of breath. He shows symptoms of which of the following respiratory diseases?
    a. Bronchitis
    b. Asthma
    c. Emphysema
    d. Bronchiectasis
17. The classification of burns that is the most painful is:
    a. First degree
    b. Second degree
    c. Third degree
    d. Fourth degree
18. A positive Thompson test would be indicative of what disorder?
    a. Anterior compartment syndrome of the calf
    b. Tarsal tunnel syndrome
    c. Ruptured Achilles tendon
    d. Torn anterior cruciate ligament
19. A patient has just been told he has a separated shoulder. His injury is in what joint?
    a. Sternoclavicular
    b. Coracoclavicular
    c. Acromioclavicular
    d. Glenohumeral
20. Gout most often involves the:
    a. Ankle joint
    b. Hip
    c. Large toe
    d. Knee
21. The top of the iliac crest is at what spinal level?
    a. L2
    b. L4
    c. T12
    d. L5
22. If a patient has a diminished biceps reflex, which spinal segment do you expect to be involved?
    a. C2
    b. C4
    c. C5-6
    d. C1-2
23. In rotator cuff tears the tendon most commonly involved is the:
    a. Infraspinatus
    b. Supraspinatus
    c. Teres minor
    d. Subscapularis
24. Impingement syndrome at the shoulder most often involves the:
    a. Biceps tendon
    b. Supraspinatus
    c. Infraspinatus
    d. a and b
    e. b and c

25. A patient complaining of tennis elbow would have the greatest pain over the:
    a. Olecranon
    b. Medial epicondyle
    c. Lateral epicondyle
    d. None of the above
26. Carpal tunnel syndrome is a compression syndrome of which nerve?
    a. Median
    b. Ulnar
    c. Radial
    d. Brachial
27. A Colles' fracture involves which bone the most?
    a. Humerus
    b. Radius
    c. Ulna
    d. Hamate
28. De Quervain's syndrome involves which tendon(s)?
    a. Abductor pollicis longus
    b. Extensor pollicis longus
    c. Flexor pollicis brevis
    d. Extensor pollicis brevis
    e. a and d
29. Piriformis syndrome involves the entrapment of which nerve?
    a. Femoral
    b. Obturator
    c. Sciatic
    d. Gluteal
30. In a positive anterior drawer test at the knee, the:
    a. Tibia moves anterior on the femur with a forward pull
    b. Femur moves anterior on the tibia with a forward pull
    c. Patella moves superior when anterior pressure is placed on the tibia
    d. None of the above
31. When a valgus stress is placed on the knee, the stress is applied on the:
    a. Anterior shin
    b. Outside or lateral side of the knee
    c. Inside the knee
    d. Medial side of the knee
32. You are seeing a patient who has been diagnosed as having chondromalacia of the knee. In most cases which muscle is weak?
    a. Rectus femoris
    b. Biceps femoris
    c. Vastus medialis obliquus
    d. Vastus lateralis
33. A disease characterized by inflammation of the brain and meninges and thought to be carried by birds and transmitted by mosquitoes is:
    a. Meningitis
    b. Poliomyelitis
    c. Encephalitis
    d. None of the above

34. A disease characterized by the "pill roller's tremor" is:
    a. Huntington's chorea
    b. Parkinson's disease
    c. Multiple sclerosis
    d. Encephalitis
35. An individual with a C5 spinal cord injury can do all of the following *except:*
    a. Elbow flexion
    b. Scapula elevation
    c. Shoulder external rotation
    d. Forearm pronation
36. A person with an L2 spinal cord injury would *not* have:
    a. Hip flexion
    b. Full trunk control
    c. Knee extension
    d. Foot dorsiflexion
37. A patient with a weak long thoracic nerve would be expected to have:
    a. Weak supraspinatus
    b. Weak pectoralis major
    c. Winging of the scapula
    d. Weak infraspinatus
38. The ape hand deformity is characteristic of an injury to which nerve?
    a. Median
    b. Radial
    c. Ulnar
    d. Musculocutaneous
39. A 59-year-old man was involved in an explosion and burned his legs badly. He will receive temporary grafts from a cadaver. These grafts are called:
    a. Autografts
    b. Allografts
    c. Homografts
    d. Xenografts
    e. b and d

REFERENCES

1. Booher JM: *Athletic injury assessment*, ed 3, St Louis, 1994, Mosby.
2. Hartley A: *Practical joint assessment: upper quadrant*, ed 2, St Louis, 1995, Mosby.

SUGGESTED READINGS

Booher JM: *Athletic injury assessment*, ed 3, St Louis, 1994, Mosby.
Hamann B: *Disease: identification, prevention, and control*, St Louis, 1994, Mosby.
Hartley A: *Practical joint assessment: lower quadrant*, ed 2, St Louis, 1995, Mosby.
Hartley A: *Practical joint assessment: upper quadrant*, ed 2, St Louis, 1995, Mosby.
Hertling D: *Management of common musculoskeletal disorders*, ed 2, Philadelphia, 1990, JB Lippincott.
Hoppenfield S: *Physical examination of the spine and extremities*, East Norwalk, Conn., 1978, Appleton & Lange.
Merck Manual, ed 12, New Jersey, 1993, Merck.
Mulvihill ML: *Human diseases*, ed 2, Los Altos, Calif., 1987, Appleton Davies.
O'Sullivan C: *Physical rehabilitation*, Philadelphia, 1981, FA Davis.
Rothstein JM: *Rehabilitation specialist's handbook*, Philadelphia, 1991, FA Davis.
Seeley RR: *Anatomy and physiology*, ed 2, St Louis, 1992, Mosby.

EXAMINATION ANSWER KEY

1.	a	**21.**	b
2.	a	**22.**	c
3.	c	**23.**	b
4.	c	**24.**	d
5.	a	**25.**	c
6.	c	**26.**	a
7.	b	**27.**	b
8.	d	**28.**	e
9.	c	**29.**	c
10.	c	**30.**	a
11.	a	**31.**	b
12.	b	**32.**	c
13.	c	**33.**	c
14.	c	**34.**	b
15.	c	**35.**	d
16.	c	**36.**	d
17.	b	**37.**	c
18.	c	**38.**	a
19.	c	**39.**	e
20.	c		

EXAMINATION ANSWER SHEET

1. _____

2. _____

3. _____

4. _____

5. _____

6. _____

7. _____

8. _____

9. _____

10. _____

11. _____

12. _____

13. _____

14. _____

15. _____

16. _____

17. _____

18. _____

19. _____

20. _____

21. _____

22. _____

23. _____

24. _____

25. _____

26. _____

27. _____

28. _____

29. _____

30. _____

31. _____

32. _____

33. _____

34. _____

35. _____

36. _____

37. _____

38. _____

39. _____

EXAMINATION ANSWER SHEET

1. _____

2. _____

3. _____

4. _____

5. _____

6. _____

7. _____

8. _____

9. _____

10. _____

11. _____

12. _____

13. _____

14. _____

15. _____

16. _____

17. _____

18. _____

19. _____

20. _____

21. _____

22. _____

23. _____

24. _____

25. _____

26. _____

27. _____

28. _____

29. _____

30. _____

31. _____

32. _____

33. _____

34. _____

35. _____

36. _____

37. _____

38. _____

39. _____

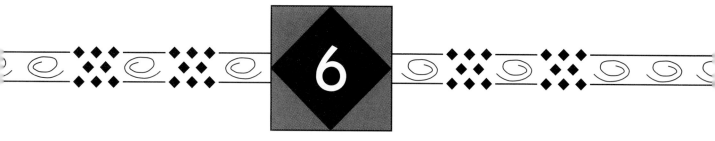

Psychological Disorders

Psychology is the branch of science that deals with the study, diagnosis, treatment, and prevention of human behavioral disorders. Psycho- logical factors contribute to many physical disorders and may appear as a reaction to a physical disorder.

COMMON PSYCHOLOGICAL DISORDERS

I. Schizophrenia is a group of psychotic disorders characterized by delusions, hallucinations, bizarre behavior, withdrawal, conflicting emotions, and flat affect (emotions). Approximately 50% of all patients in mental hospitals have schizophrenia.
   A. Personality
      1. As a child, the schizophrenic patient was quiet, obedient, and passive and did not form friendships.
      2. As an adolescent, the schizophrenic patient is introverted, daydreams, and avoids social activities.
      3. Somatic symptoms such as stomach disorders, headaches, back or neck pain may be present.
   B. Thought disorders
      1. Disorders of content include the idea that someone is controlling your thoughts and the idea that people are talking about you.
      2. Disorders of form of thoughts
         a) *Word mix:* incoherent, unrelated combination of words
         b) *Loose association:* shifting of ideas from one subject to another in an unrelated fashion during conversation
         c) *Neologisms:* newly formed words whose meaning is known only to person who is using them
         d) *Echolalia:* repetition of a word over and over again
      3. Disorders of thought process include short attention span, abrupt halt in the train of thought, impaired memory, and lack of abstract thinking. Although thought disorders are most common in schizophrenia, they also occur with other psychological disorders (e.g., mania).
   C. Suicide in patients with schizophrenia is common. More than 50% attempt suicide.
   D. Etiology: among the many theories as to the cause of schizophrenia are:
      1. Poor organization of the ego

2. Poor input in decision making from parents. According to this theory, the child constantly receives contradictory information from the parents, making decision making on the part of the child impossible.
3. Dysfunctional neurotransmission system
   a) Dopamine hypothesis: some researchers believe that the dopaminergic system is hyperactive in schizophrenic patients.
   b) Norepinephrine activity also may be elevated.
  E. Schizophrenia most often manifests in middle age.
II. Conversion disorder (hysterical neurosis) is a neurotic disorder characterized by numerous somatic symptoms for which there are no organic causes.
III. Mania is an emotional state characterized by elevated mood and hyperactivity, lack of inhibition, talkativeness, and impulsivity.
IV. Depression is an emotional state characterized by diminished interest in usual activities, reduced energy, decreased motivation, impaired thinking, and weight loss. Typically a person does not have enough energy to commit suicide while severely depressed; however, the risk of suicide increases once the depression lessens. Untreated depression lasts 6 to 12 months; treated depression lasts about 3 months.
V. Hypochondriasis is a disorder characterized by the preoccupation with one's bodily functions and the obsession that one is suffering from a serious disease.
VI. Acrophobia is a common disorder involving the fear of heights.

REVIEW QUESTIONS

1. Which of the following is believed to be the main neurotransmitter involved in schizophrenia?
   a. Acetylcholine
   b. Dopamine
   c. Endorphins
   d. Norepinephrine
   e. Enkephalin
2. The percentage of people with schizophrenia who attempt suicide is about:
   a. 10%
   b. 20%
   c. 30%
   d. 50%
   e. 75%
3. A 15 year-old-boy who had his first schizophrenic episode in 6 months will be least likely to show:
   a. Abnormal mood changes
   b. Strange behavior
   c. Strange perceptions
   d. Excessive spending
   e. Somatic complaints
4. Which of the following symptoms is *least* likely to occur in an individual experiencing a manic episode?
   a. Loose association
   b. Flight of ideas
   c. Word mix
   d. Neologisms
   e. Lack of energy

5. Which of the following is characteristic of a depression disorder?
   a. Severely depressed people often do not have the energy to commit suicide
   b. As depression lessens, the risk of suicide decreases
   c. Orientation to person, place, and time is usually impaired
   d. Presence of delusions indicates that the individual is schizophrenic, not depressed
6. Which of the following terms is used for someone who is afraid of heights?
   a. Acrophobia
   b. Altiphobia
   c. Milaphobia
   d. Algaphobia
7. Which of the following does *not* apply to schizophrenia?
   a. It usually begins in middle age
   b. There is a separation from reality
   c. The onset may be either gradual or sudden
   d. In childhood, patients are quiet, passive, and obedient
8. Which of the following is true about depression?
   a. It usually will resolve in 1 to 2 weeks with treatment
   b. It is a disturbance of the dopamine system
   c. It is characterized by reduced energy, lack of motivation, and weight loss
   d. It is characterized by making up new words
9. *Echolalia* is defined as:
   a. Making up new words
   b. Speaking with unrelated words
   c. Repeating the same word over and over
   d. Shifting of ideas from one topic to another in an unrelated fashion
10. About what percentage of patients in mental hospitals suffer from schizophrenia?
    a. 10%
    b. 15% to 20%
    c. 20% to 30%
    d. 30% to 40%
    e. 40% to 50%

SUGGESTED READINGS

Fadem B: *Behavioral science,* ed 2, Philadelphia, 1994, Harwal.
Merck Manual, ed 16, New Jersey, 1991, Merck.

EXAMINATION ANSWER KEY

1. b
2. d
3. d
4. e
5. a
6. a
7. a
8. c
9. c
10. e

EXAMINATION ANSWER SHEET

1. _____

2. _____

3. _____

4. _____

5. _____

6. _____

7. _____

8. _____

9. _____

10. _____

EXAMINATION ANSWER SHEET

1. _____

2. _____

3. _____

4. _____

5. _____

6. _____

7. _____

8. _____

9. _____

10. _____

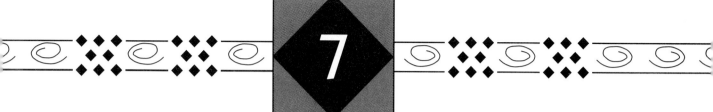

Pediatric Growth and Development

A thorough neurological examination is extremely important in evaluating and diagnosing disorders of the pediatric musculoskeletal system. Such an evaluation is especially vital when muscle weakness or diminished neuromuscular function is suspected in a newborn. It is also important to be familiar with the normal pediatric sequence of motor skill development.

NEUROLOGICAL REFLEX ASSESSMENT

Reflex	Action	Age of Integration
Grasp	When pencil is placed in ulnar side of palm, the fingers close around it	4 to 6 months
Moro	Sudden startle reaction in which all four extremities abduct and extend and spine extends	5 to 6 months
Startle	Flexion of elbows and clenching of fingers caused by sudden loud noise or tapping on sternum	Persists in adult
Flexor withdrawal	Dorsiflexion of ankle and flexion of hip and knee in response to pinstick to sole of foot	1 to 2 months
Asymmetrical tonic neck	Rotation of head to one side causes arm on rotated side to extend	4 to 6 months
Symmetrical tonic neck	Flexion of head causes flexion of arms and extension of legs; extension of head causes extension of arms and flexion of legs	8 to 12 months
Landau	When infant is held in prone position with support under thorax, the neck, spine, and hips extend	4 months
Neck righting	When infant is supine with head in midline and then head is rotated to one side, the body turns as a whole to same side	6 months
Body righting	When infant is supine and upper or lower trunk is rotated, the extremities follow	6 to 18 months
Labyrinthine righting	If infant is placed in prone position, vision is blocked, and body position is altered by tilting infant in different positions, the infant will always raise head to normal position with mouth horizontal	Persists in adult
Rooting reflex	When side of cheek or upper or lower lip is stimulated, the infant will turn mouth and face toward stimulus	3 to 4 months
Visual tracking	Infant follows moving object with eyes	1 to 3 months

MOTOR DEVELOPMENT

Developmental age	Skill
1 to 3 months	Voluntary movement of arms from midline, focusing, visual tracking, grasp reflex
3 to 6 months	Lifts head from prone position, brings hands to midline, extends back from supine position (bridging), rolls from prone to supine position, vocalizes without crying, pulls to sitting position, moves objects from one hand to the other, does not exhibit extensor lag of head when pulled from supine to sitting position
6 to 9 months	Reaches out and touches objects, sits without support, turns head side to side, brings hand to mouth for feeding, laughs and smiles, pulls to standing position, crawls (at 9 months can feed finger foods to self)
12 months	Leans and recovers balance when sitting, walks (may require one-hand support), goes up and down stairs, attempts to stack blocks, bangs two objects together, rolls ball, picks up spoon, begins speaking two words
14 months	Stands without support, walks forward, stoops and recovers balance, eats food alone, drinks out of cup, begins to assist in dressing
18 months	Turns pages, puts pegs in holes, walks sideways and backward, steps up and down small elevations, walks faster
2 years	Ascends stairs without support, runs forward, kicks ball, demonstrates increased dressing skills, feeds self with spoon
3 years	Jumps in place, rides tricycle, walks heel to toe
4 years	Balances on one foot, runs, throws overhand, puts shoes on right feet, brushes hair and teeth
5 years	Hops, catches ball, jumps off object and lands on two feet
School age	Handedness is normally established

REVIEW QUESTIONS

1. You are working with a child on the mat and notice that he attempts to reach for a toy, is able to maintain good alignment when you pull him to sitting, and can roll from prone to supine position. What age would you expect this child to be?
   a. 8 months
   b. 5 months
   c. 7 months
   d. 9 months

2. Which of the following would you *not* expect to occur before an infant is 6 months of age, assuming normal development?
   a. Rolling from prone to supine position
   b. Bringing hand to mouth for feeding
   c. Bringing hands to midline
   d. Pulling to sitting position

3. At which age would you expect a child to be able to pull to standing?
   a. 3 months
   b. 7 months
   c. 11 months
   d. 10 months

4. By which age should a child be able to sit without support?
   a. 7 months
   b. 4 months
   c. 10 months
   d. 12 months

5. You are working with a 3-month-old infant and a sudden movement elicits a startle reaction. This is characteristic of what reflex?
   a. Grasp
   b. Tonic neck
   c. Extensor
   d. Moro
6. Failure to dorsiflex and pull the foot away after the foot is pricked with a pin would be a negative response for which reflex?
   a. Moro
   b. Babinski
   c. Flexor withdrawal
   d. Labyrinthine
7. The asymmetrical tonic neck reflex is characterized by which of the following?
   a. Flexion of the head with resultant flexion of the arms and extension of the legs
   b. Flexion of the neck with resultant flexion of the arms and legs
   c. Rotation of the head with resultant extension of the arm on the rotated side
   d. Extension of the neck with resultant extension of the arms and legs
8. A 12-month-old infant should be able to do all of the following *except:*
   a. Walk with one-hand support
   b. Go up and down stairs
   c. Walk sideways and backwards
   d. Attempt to stack blocks
9. Which of the following skills does *not* normally develop between the ninth and twelfth months of age?
   a. Pulling to standing
   b. Jumping in place
   c. Attempting to stack blocks
   d. Rolling a ball
10. Stroking the right cheek of an infant will cause her to turn her mouth to the right. This is an example of which reflex?
    a. Moro
    b. Labyrinthine righting
    c. Rooting
    d. Righting
11. The presence of a symmetrical tonic neck reflex is seen when:
    a. Rotation of the head to the side causes the legs to flex
    b. Lateral flexion of the neck causes the arm on the same side to flex
    c. Rotation of the head to the side causes the arm on the same side to extend
    d. Flexion of the head causes flexion of the arms and extension of the legs
12. You are working with a 4-month-old infant, who is supine on the mat. When you rotate her head to one side, the body turns as a whole to the same side. This is evidence of which reflex?
    a. Landau
    b. Neck righting
    c. Body righting
    d. Labyrinthine righting

13. Handedness is normally established by the age of:
    a. 2 years
    b. 3 years
    c. School age
    d. 10 years
14. Visual tracking is which of the following?
    a. Ability to follow a moving object with the eyes
    b. Ability to remember a previously seen visual image
    c. Inability to judge the distance of a moving object
    d. Disorder involving the inability to determine the speed at which an object is moving

SUGGESTED READINGS

Chusid J: *Correlative neuroanatomy,* Los Altos, 1987, Lange Medical Publications.
Merck Manual, ed 16, New Jersey, 1992, Merck.
Rothstein JM: *Rehabilitation specialist's handbook,* Philadelphia, 1991, FA Davis.
Tachdjian MO: *Pediatric orthopedics,* Philadelphia, 1972, WB Saunders.

EXAMINATION ANSWER KEY

1. b
2. b
3. b
4. a
5. d
6. c
7. c
8. c
9. b
10. c
11. d
12. b
13. c
14. a

EXAMINATION ANSWER SHEET

1. _____

2. _____

3. _____

4. _____

5. _____

6. _____

7. _____

8. _____

9. _____

10. _____

11. _____

12. _____

13. _____

14. _____

EXAMINATION ANSWER SHEET

1. _____

2. _____

3. _____

4. _____

5. _____

6. _____

7. _____

8. _____

9. _____

10. _____

11. _____

12. _____

13. _____

14. _____

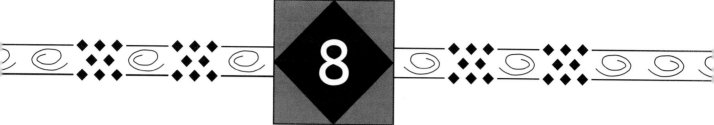

Physical Therapy Modalities and Procedures

Controversy over the role and use of physical therapy modalities and procedures is not new. Unfortunately these modalities have been applied in a very passive, mechanical manner. There is no question, however, that modalities or physical agents are useful tools in the effective treatment and rehabilitation of patients with musculoskeletal pain and dysfunction. Modalities include a long list of techniques and devices or machines to administer heat, cold, sound, light, water, and electricity. Under no circumstance should passive modalities be used as a total treatment. They should be used instead in combination with other procedures after proper assessment and evaluation to promote healing and/or rehabilitation. This chapter describes the most common modalities and procedures used in physical therapy clinics.

COMMON MODALITIES

Modalities may be divided into the following basic types: (1) cryotherapy (cold), (2) thermotherapy (heat), and (3) electrical stimulation.

I. Infrared modalities—Of all the modalities discussed in this chapter, the most frequently used are those classified as infrared modalities in the electromagnetic spectrum. Infrared energy falls between microwave diathermy and the visible light portions of the spectrum. The modalities included in the infrared spectrum are moist hot packs, heating pads, whirlpools, infrared lamps, and paraffin baths. All of these various classifications of radiation comprise the electromagnetic spectrum.[3] The decision of which modality to use depends on the shape and size of the area to be treated, depth of the tissue involved, convenience of the modality, and absence of contraindications.
   A. Indications
      1. Soft tissue injuries
      2. When patient cannot tolerate weight of hot pack
   B. Contraindications
      1. Acute inflammatory condition
      2. Fever
      3. Active bleeding
      4. Cardiac problems
      5. Decreased circulation

C. Cryotherapy (cold) is the local application of cold to gain therapeutic results.
   1. Application methods
      a) Ice packs (Fig. 8-1)
      b) Ice massage (Fig. 8-2)
      c) Contrast bath
      d) Vapocoolant spray
      e) Iced towels
      f) Cold baths or whirlpools (Fig. 8-3)
   2. Indications
      a) Swelling in acute musculoskeletal injuries
      b) Spasticity in central nervous system (CNS) disorders
      c) Postoperative swelling
      d) Burns (emergency care)
      e) Inflammation (acute treatment)
      f) Fever
   3. Contraindications
      a) Raynaud's phenomenon
      b) Cardiac or respiratory disorders
      c) Open wounds
      d) Hypersensitivity to cold
      e) Decreased sensation and/or arterial insufficiency
      f) Angina pectoris
   4. Physiological effects
      a) Local vasoconstriction
      b) Slowing down of nerve conduction velocity
      c) Decrease in muscle spasticity
      d) Decrease in inflammation
      e) Decrease in and limitation of hemorrhage

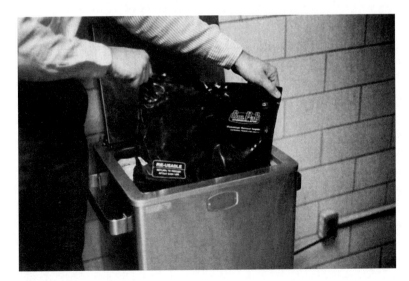

FIG. 8-1. Commercial ice packs. (From Prentice WE: *Therapeutic modalities in sports medicine*, St Louis, 1986, Mosby.)

f) Decrease in swelling and edema
g) Analgesia
h) Decrease in respiratory and heart rate
i) Change in local sensation from a sensation of cold, burning, aching, and finally numbness[1]

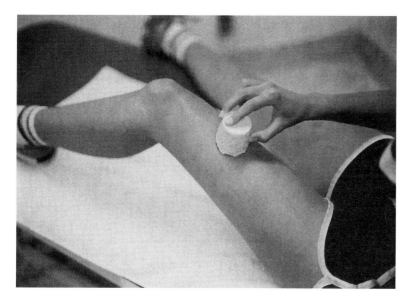

FIG. 8-2.   Ice massage. (From Prentice WE: *Therapeutic modalities in sports medicine,* St Louis, 1986, Mosby.)

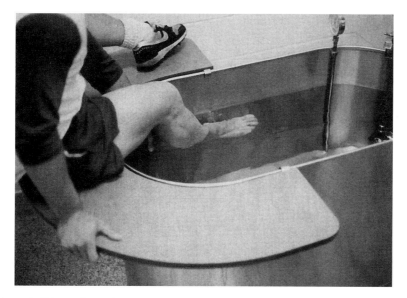

IG. 8-3.   Cold whirlpool. (From Prentice WE: *Therapeutic modalities in sports medicine,* St Louis, 1986, Mosby.)

D. Thermotherapy (heat)
1. Application methods[1]
   a) *Conduction:* transfer of heat by direct contact with its source (e.g., hot packs or paraffin)
   b) *Convection:* transfer of heat by a medium of air or water (e.g., whirlpool)
   c) *Radiation:* transfer of heat or energy through space by electromagnetic waves (e.g., infrared)
   d) *Conversion:* production of heat by the passing of sound or electric current through the tissue of the body (e.g., ultrasound and diathermy)
2. Physiological effects
   a) Decrease in pain
   b) Decrease in muscle spasm
   c) Increase in cell metabolism
   d) Increase in range of motion when used in combination with stretching
   e) Increase in blood flow, which leads to removal of waste products in injured area
3. Types of thermotherapy
   a) Superficial thermotherapy
      (1) Whirlpool (Fig. 8-4)
         (a) Indications
            i) Wound care
            ii) Burns
            iii) Diminished circulation
            iv) Swelling
            v) Subacute or chronic inflammation
            vi) Range of motion deficit
         (b) Contraindications
            i) Infection
            ii) Fever

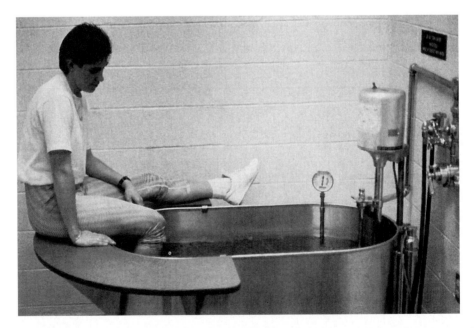

FIG. 8-4. Warm whirlpool. (From Prentice WE: *Therapeutic modalities in sports medicine,* St Louis, 1986, Mosby.)

   iii) Circulatory disorders

   iv) Acute inflammatory conditions

   v) Bleeding

  (c) Water temperatures in whirlpools

	Temperature	
Description[2]	**Fahrenheit (°F)**	**Centigrade (°C)**
Very hot	104-110	40-43.5
Hot	99-104	37-40
Warm	96-99	35.5-37
Neutral	92-96	33.5-35.5
Tepid	80-92	27-33.5

(2) Hydrocollator (hot) packs (Fig. 8-5) are immersed in 160° to 170° F water.

  (a) Indications

   i) Muscle spasm

   ii) Pain

   iii) Diminished range of motion

  (b) Contraindications

   i) Acute inflammatory conditions

   ii) Decreased circulation or sensation

   iii) Malignancy

   iv) Active bleeding

   v) Cardiac insufficiency

   vi) Open wounds

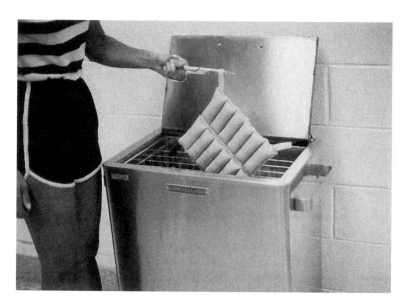

FIG. 8-5. Hydrocollator (hot) packs. (From Prentice WE: *Therapeutic modalities in sports medicine,* St Louis, 1986, Mosby.)

    (3) Paraffin bath (Fig. 8-6) requires that the paraffin is melted and used at 125° to 130° F.

        (a) Indications

            i) Joint injuries

            ii) Subacute or chronic inflammatory conditions

        (b) Contraindications

            i) Open wounds

            ii) Decreased circulation

            iii) Acute inflammation

    (4) Fluidotherapy (Fig. 8-7) involves the use of the fluidotherapy unit, a dry heat modality that uses a suspended air stream, which has the properties of a liquid. Its therapeutic usefulness in rehabilitation and healing is due to its ability to apply heat, massage, sensory stimulation, and levitation at the same time.[3]

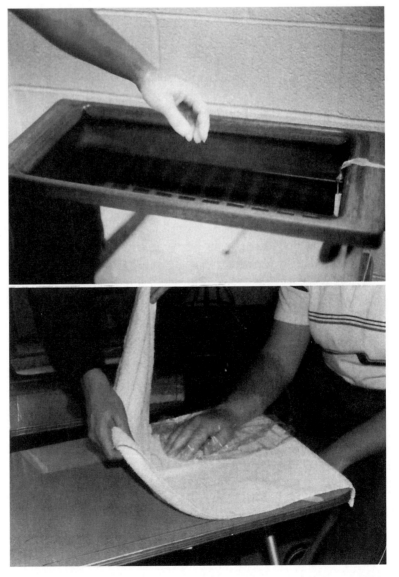

FIG. 8-6. Paraffin bath. (From Prentice WE: *Therapeutic modalities in sports medicine,* St Louis, 1986, Mosby.)

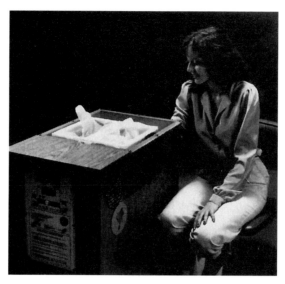

FIG. 8-7.   Fluidotherapy. (From Prentice WE: *Therapeutic modalities in sports medicine,* St Louis, 1986, Mosby.)

    (a) Indications
        i) Pain
        ii) Diminished range of motion
        iii) Swelling
        iv) Wound healing
        v) Diminished circulation
    (b) Contraindications
        i) Infections
        ii) Diminished sensation
  b) Penetrating thermotherapy penetrates 2 inches (5 cm).
    (1) Diathermy produces heat by converting high-frequency electromagnetic energy to heat energy in the patient's connective tissue. *Short-wave diathermy* generators produce high-frequency electromagnetic waves with a length of 11 m and a frequency of 27 MHz.[4]
      (a) Indications
        i) Diminished circulation
        ii) Muscle spasm
        iii) Pain
        iv) Muscle strain
      (b) Contraindications
        i) Bleeding
        ii) Pacemakers
        iii) Malignancy
        iv) Metal implants
        v) Pregnancy
        vi) Infection
        vii) Acute inflammation
        viii) Cardiac disease

(2) Ultraviolet radiation is radiant energy in the wavelength band of 180 to 400 nanometers (nm). This band is further divided into three bands[2]:

Band	Wavelength
UVA	320-400 nm
UVB	290-320 nm
UVC	180-290 nm

Two major types of generators produce ultraviolet radiation. The air-cooled, high-pressure mercury vapor lamp is one of the most common generators. It consists of a quartz tube that transmits ultraviolet waves. Within the quartz tube is argon gas into which mercury is placed. These generators operate at high temperatures and are cooled by circulating air; therefore they are called *hot quartz generators.*[2] The other type of generator, a *cold quartz generator,* operates in a manner very similar to that of the hot quartz generator. Its output is limited to the UVC band. Due to its small size and low heat output, it is portable and easy to use at the bedside.[2]

- **(a)** Indications
    - **i)** Acne
    - **ii)** Wounds or pressure sores
    - **iii)** Psoriasis
    - **iv)** Septic wounds
- **(b)** Contraindications
    - **i)** Decreased circulation
    - **ii)** Regimen of medication that may cause increased sensitivity to ultraviolet light
    - **iii)** New skin grafts or scars
    - **iv)** Lupus erythematosus
    - **v)** Severe diabetes
    - **vi)** Severe heart conditions
- **(c)** Physiological effects
    - **i)** Vasodilation
    - **ii)** Activation of steroids
    - **iii)** Vasomotor stimulation
    - **iv)** Analgesia to nerve endings
    - **v)** Increased muscle tone
    - **vi)** Stimulation of metabolism
    - **vii)** Possible sterilization qualities
    - **viii)** Psychological benefits

(3) Ultrasound is the name given to sound waves produced by a crystal located within a transducer or soundhead. The sound waves are produced as the crystal vibrates. The frequency for ultrasound is 800,000 to 3,000,000 Hz (0.8 to 3 MHz).
- **(a)** Indications
    - **i)** Shortened tissue (e.g., contractures, scar tissue)
    - **ii)** Plantar warts
    - **iii)** Diminished circulation
    - **iv)** Muscle spasm
    - **v)** Subacute or chronic inflammation

         (b) Contraindications
- **i)** Poor arterial supply
- **ii)** Open wounds
- **iii)** Cancer
- **iv)** Pregnancy (especially use of ultrasound over low back or uterus)
- **v)** Use over eyes
- **vi)** Use over heart or in the presence of a pacemaker
- **vii)** Decreased circulation
- **viii)** Use over spinal cord
- **ix)** Use over carotid sinus

    (c) Physiological effects: same as those for ultraviolet radiation

II. Electrical stimulation
- **A.** Transcutaneous electrical nerve stimulation (TENS) is a method of afferent stimulation developed to control pain. TENS is based on the work of Melzack and Wall.[5] Their theory suggests that the peripheral stimulation of large-diameter cutaneous afferent nerve fibers can block pain sensation at the spinal cord, preventing it from reaching the conscious brain.[4] The various modes of TENS are identified by their parameter ranges of amplitude, frequency, and pulse width.[2]
  - **1.** Indications
    - *a)* Pain
    - *b)* Hypersensitive trigger points
    - *c)* Muscle spasm
  - **2.** Contraindications
    - *a)* Pacemaker
    - *b)* Severe cardiac problems
    - *c)* Open wounds
    - *d)* Thrombophlebitis
    - *e)* Use near the heart
    - *f)* Malignancy
- **B.** High-voltage stimulation is stimulation provided by a device using a voltage greater than 150 volts at a medium frequency. High-voltage stimulation uses a twin-peaked, monophasic current and produces between 150 and 500 volts.
  - **1.** Indications
    - *a)* Pain
    - *b)* Hypersensitive trigger points
    - *c)* Muscle spasm
    - *d)* Diminished blood flow
  - **2.** Contraindications: same as those for TENS
  - **3.** Physiological effect
    - *a)* Tissue healing
- **C.** Low-voltage stimulation allows the use of either biphasic or monophasic current and usually delivers between 0 and 150 volts.[1]
- **D.** Iontophoresis uses galvanic (DC) current to drive or introduce selected ions into body tissues.
  - **1.** Indications
    - *a)* Swelling
    - *b)* Muscle spasm
    - *c)* Hypersensitive trigger points
    - *d)* Inflammation
    - *e)* Bursitis

        f) Decubitus ulcers

        g) Plantar warts

        h) Certain fungus infections

    2. Contraindications: same as those for TENS

E. Inferential stimulation uses two biphasic medium-frequency currents between 4000 and 5000 cycles/sec. The higher frequencies are used to lower tissue resistance, thereby causing a stronger response with less current intensity.

COMMON PROCEDURES

I. Massage is one of the oldest physical therapy procedures recorded. Massage is defined as the mechanical stimulation of the tissue by means of rhythmically applied pressure and stretching.[3] Several different strokes can be used in massage.

  A. Most common types of massage strokes

    1. Effleurage is a stroke that glides over the skin lightly without attempting to move the deep muscle tissues. The main purpose of effleurage is to help the patient to adjust to the physical contact with the therapist's or assistant's hands.[3] Every massage begins and ends with effleurage strokes.

    2. Petrissage consists of kneading manipulation that presses and rolls the muscles under the therapist's or assistant's fingers. The purpose of petrissage is to increase venous and lymphatic return, break up adhesions, loosen adherent fibrous tissue, and increase the elasticity of the skin.[3]

    3. Friction is the type of massage James Cyriax has used to affect musculoskeletal structures of ligament, tendon, and muscle to provide therapeutic movement over a small area. The purpose of friction massage is to loosen adhesions, increase the absorption of edema, and reduce muscle spasm.

    4. Percussion or tapotement massage consists of a series of quick blows, given with the relaxed hands, that follow each other in rapid sequence. Percussion is used to stimulate subcutaneous structures. There are several types of percussion massage:

        a) *Hacking:* alternate striking of the patient with the ulnar border of the hand

        b) *Slapping:* alternate slapping with the fingers

        c) *Beating:* striking with half-closed fist using the hypothenar eminence of the hand

        d) *Tapping:* striking with the tips of the fingers

        e) *Clapping or cupping:* percussion massage used primarily in postural drainage[3]

  B. Indications

    1. Diminished circulation

    2. Swelling

    3. Muscle spasm

    4. Tight scar tissue

    5. Diminished circulation

  C. Contraindications

    1. Injuries with hemorrhaging

    2. Infection

    3. Thrombophlebitis

    4. Malignancy

II. Mechanical traction involves the use of electronic traction machines to exert a gentle pull or force through a rope attached to halters and straps.

A. Indications
   1. Pain
   2. Muscle spasm
   3. Realignment of spine
   4. Herniated disc
   5. Facet joint symptoms
B. Contraindications
   1. Spinal fractures
   2. Severe segmental instability
   3. Tumors in traction area
   4. Acute disc herniation
   5. Pregnancy
C. Physiological effects
   1. Separation of vertebral segments
   2. Distraction of the facet joints
   3. Stretching of the spinal muscles

III. Goniometry is the measurement of the range of motion of joints. The following text outlines the movements, axes, goniometer arm placement, positions of testing, and normal ranges of motions (in parentheses) according to Sinaki.[6]

A. Shoulder
   1. Flexion (180 degrees)/extension (45 degrees) (Fig. 8-8)
      a) Axis: center of the shoulder joint on the lateral side
      b) Position: supine
      c) Stationary arm: midline of the trunk (axillary line)
      d) Movable arm: midline of the shaft of the humerus (lateral side)

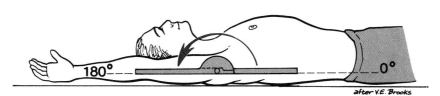

FIG. 8-8. Shoulder flexion. (From Erickson RP, McPhee MC: Clinical evaluation. In DeLisa JA, editor: *Rehabilitation medicine: principles and practice,* ed 2, Philadelphia, 1993, JB Lippincott.)

   2. Abduction (180 degrees)/adduction (30 degrees) (Fig. 8-9)
      a) Axis: center of the shoulder joint on the posterior side
      b) Position: sitting
      c) Stationary arm: parallel to the longitudinal axis or midline of the back
      d) Movable arm: midline of the shaft of the humerus
   3. Internal (70 degrees)/external (90 degrees) rotation (Figs. 8-10 and 8-11)
      a) Axis: olecranon process
      b) Position: supine
      c) Stationary arm: perpendicular or parallel to the trunk
      d) Movable arm: midline between the shaft of the ulna and the styloid process

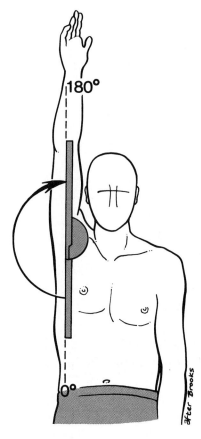

FIG. 8-9.   Shoulder abduction. (From Erickson RP, McPhee MC: Clinical evaluation. In DeLisa JA, editor: *Rehabilitation medicine: principles and practice,* ed 2, Philadelphia, 1993, JB Lippincott.)

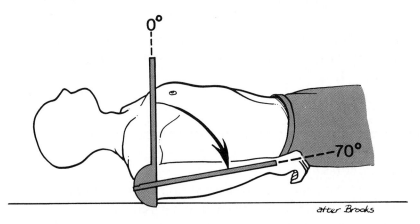

FIG. 8-10.   Shoulder internal rotation. (From Erickson RP, McPhee MC: Clinical evaluation. In DeLisa JA, editor: *Rehabilitation medicine: principles and practice,* ed 2, Philadelphia, 1993, JB Lippincott.)

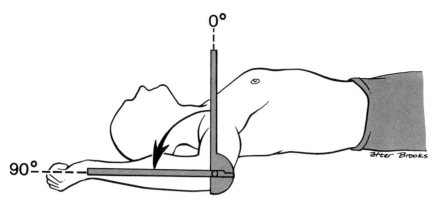

FIG. 8-11.   Shoulder external rotation. (From Erickson RP, McPhee MC: Clinical evaluation. In DeLisa JA, editor: *Rehabilitation medicine: principles and practice,* ed 2, Philadelphia, 1993, JB Lippincott.)

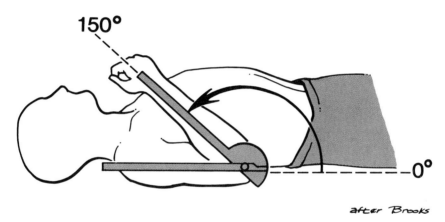

FIG. 8-12.   Elbow flexion. (From Erickson RP, McPhee MC: Clinical evaluation. In DeLisa JA, editor: *Rehabilitation medicine: principles and practice,* ed 2, Philadelphia, 1993, JB Lippincott.)

    4. Horizontal abduction/adduction
        a) Axis: superior on the acromion process
        b) Position: sitting
        c) Stationary arm: horizontal or perpendicular to the trunk
        d) Movable arm: midline of the shaft of the humerus
  B. Elbow
    1. Flexion (150 degrees)/extension (Fig. 8-12)
        a) Axis: lateral epicondyle of the humerus
        b) Position: supine
        c) Stationary arm: lateral midline of the humerus
        d) Movable arm: lateral midline of the ulna
    2. Pronation (80 degrees)/supination (80 degrees) (Figs. 8-13 and 8-14)
        a) Axis: styloid process of the ulna
        b) Position: sitting
        c) Stationary arm: anterior and parallel to the midline of the humerus
        d) Movable arm: supination—palmar surface of the wrist
                         pronation—dorsal surface of the wrist

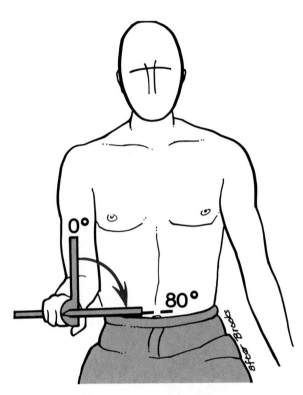

FIG. 8-13. Forearm pronation. (From Erickson RP, McPhee MC: Clinical evaluation. In DeLisa JA, editor: *Rehabilitation medicine: principles and practice,* ed 2, Philadelphia, 1993, JB Lippincott.)

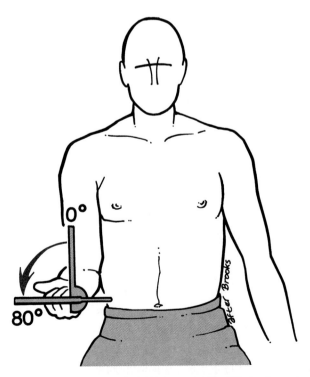

FIG. 8-14. Forearm supination. (From Erickson RP, McPhee MC: Clinical evaluation. In DeLisa JA, editor: *Rehabilitation medicine: principles and practice,* ed 2, Philadelphia, 1993, JB Lippincott.)

C. Wrist
   1. Flexion (80 degrees)/extension (70 degrees)
      a) Axis: lateral side over the styloid process
      b) Position: sitting
      c) Stationary arm: parallel to the shaft of the ulna
      d) Movable arm: midline shaft of fifth metacarpal
   2. Radial (20 degrees)/ulnar (35 degrees) deviation
      a) Axis: base of the third metacarpal
      b) Position: sitting
      c) Stationary arm: midline forearm
      d) Movable arm: midline along the third metacarpal
D. Hip
   1. Flexion (120 degrees)/extension (80 degrees) (Fig. 8-15)
      a) Axis: greater trochanter of the femur
      b) Position: supine
      c) Stationary arm: parallel to the lateral midline of the trunk
      d) Movable arm: parallel to the shaft of the femur
   2. Abduction (45 degrees)/adduction (10 degrees) (Fig. 8-16)
      a) Axis: anterior on the anterior superior iliac spine
      b) Position: supine
      c) Stationary arm: horizontal across both anterior superior iliac spines
      d) Movable arm: parallel to the shaft of the femur
   3. Internal (35 degrees)/external (45 degrees) rotation (hip and knee flexed) (Fig. 8-17)
      a) Axis: anteriorly over the center of the patella
      b) Position: supine
      c) Stationary arm: perpendicular to the floor
      d) Movable arm: midline of the tibia
E. Knee
   1. Flexion (135 degrees)/extension (Fig. 8-18)
      a) Axis: lateral over the midline
      b) Position: prone
      c) Stationary arm: aligned with the shaft of the femur
      d) Movable arm: aligned with the shaft of the fibula

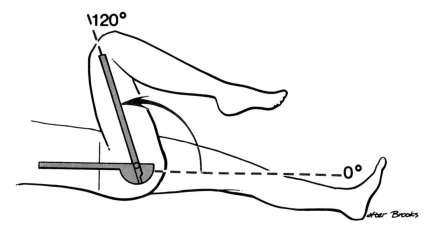

1G. 8-15.   Hip flexion. (From Erickson RP, McPhee MC: Clinical evaluation. In DeLisa JA, editor: *?ehabilitation medicine: principles and practice,* ed 2, Philadelphia, 1993, JB Lippincott.)

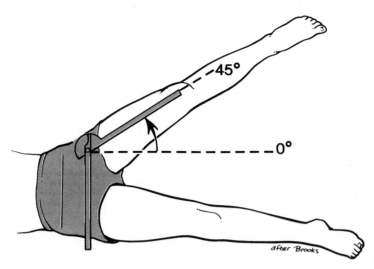

FIG. 8-16. Hip abduction. (From Erickson RP, McPhee MC: Clinical evaluation. In DeLisa JA, editor: *Rehabilitation medicine: principles and practice,* ed 2, Philadelphia, 1993, JB Lippincott.)

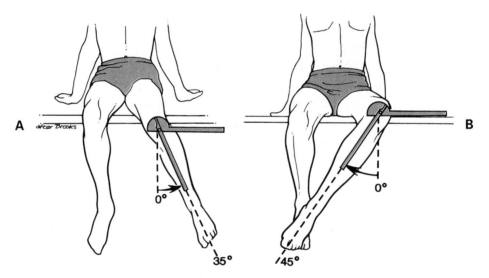

FIG. 8-17. **A,** Hip internal rotation. **B,** Hip external rotation. (From Erickson RP, McPhee MC: Clinical evaluation. In DeLisa JA, editor: *Rehabilitation medicine: principles and practice,* ed 2, Philadelphia, 1993, JB Lippincott.)

    F. Ankle
        1. Dorsiflexion (20 degrees)/plantar flexion (45 degrees) (Fig. 8-19)
            a) Axis: just inferior to lateral malleolus
            b) Position: sitting
            c) Stationary arm: midline shaft of the fibula
            d) Movable arm: midline shaft of the fifth metatarsal
        2. Eversion (20 degrees)/inversion (35 degrees)
            a) Axis: inversion—lateral side of the head of the fifth metatarsal
                eversion—medially over the head of the first metatarsal
            b) Position: sitting
            c) Stationary arm: parallel to midline of the tibia
            d) Movable arm: plantar surface over the metatarsal arch

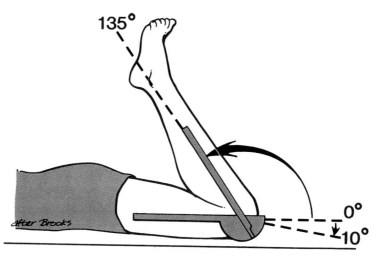

FIG. 8-18. Knee flexion. (From Erickson RP, McPhee MC: Clinical evaluation. In DeLisa JA, editor: *Rehabilitation medicine: principles and practice,* ed 2, Philadelphia, 1993, JB Lippincott.)

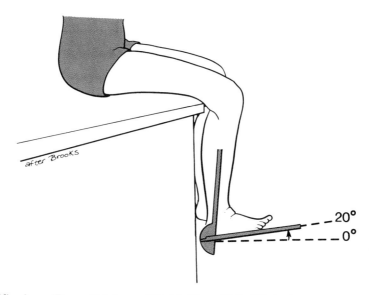

FIG. 8-19. Ankle dorsiflexion. (From Erickson RP, McPhee MC: Clinical evaluation. In DeLisa JA, editor: *Rehabilitation medicine: principles and practice,* ed 2, Philadelphia, 1993, JB Lippincott.)

IV. Muscle testing[4,6,7]

Grade		Description
6	Above normal	Ability to perform full range of motion against gravity and maximum resistance (>100%)
5	Normal	Ability to perform full range of motion against gravity and considerable resistance (100%)
4	Good	Ability to perform full range of motion against moderate resistance (80%)
3	Fair	Ability to perform full range of motion against gravity without resistance (50%)
2	Poor	Ability to perform full range of motion when gravity is eliminated (30% to 20%)
1	Trace	Ability to perform a muscle contraction that can be palpated but there is no joint motion (5%)
0	Zero	No palpable muscle contraction is demonstrated

REVIEW QUESTIONS

1. You are measuring the range of motion of a 24-year-old patient with a rotator cuff injury. When shoulder flexion is measured, the stationary arm is lined up with the:
   a. Humerus
   b. Radius
   c. Ulna
   d. Trunk
2. When TENS is being considered as a treatment modality, which of the following would *not* be a contraindication?
   a. Pacemaker
   b. Malignancy
   c. Open wound
   d. Labor pains
3. Which of the following goniometry measurements would *not* be taken with the patient sitting?
   a. Shoulder abduction
   b. Wrist extension
   c. Knee extension
   d. Forearm supination
4. The recommended position to test the strength of the rhomboid muscles is:
   a. Supine
   b. Prone
   c. Side lying
   d. Sitting
5. To measure radial deviation on the right hand of a patient, you would line the movable arm up:
   a. With the ulna
   b. With the radius
   c. With the midline of the forearm
   d. Along the third metacarpal
6. You are reviewing the chart of a patient that another assistant saw 2 days ago. When she measured pronation, she recorded 105 degrees. You would consider this motion:
   a. Normal
   b. Hypomobile
   c. Hypermobile
   d. A sign of too much stretching
7. When external rotation of the hip is measured, the stationary arm should be positioned:
   a. Parallel to the treatment table
   b. Longitudinal to the tibia
   c. Perpendicular to the floor
   d. Parallel to the midline of the femur
8. You have just reviewed the results of a muscle test performed by the physical therapist with whom you are working. He noted that the patient was able to complete 50% shoulder abduction with gravity eliminated. The muscle testing grade should be:
   a. Fair
   b. Fair minus
   c. Poor
   d. Poor minus

9. Which of the following modalities would be contraindicated for a 15-year-old boy who has an acute (<24 hours) injury to the supraspinatus tendon?
   a. Ice
   b. TENS
   c. Ultrasound
   d. Gentle massage

10. For which of the following conditions is TENS contraindicated?
    a. Use around the carotid sinus
    b. Arthritic knee
    c. Swollen ankle
    d. Fused low back

11. Which of the following is *not* a contraindication for the use of pelvic traction?
    a. Acute disc herniation
    b. Pregnancy
    c. Tumor in pelvic area
    d. Back injury 1 month postinjury

12. You are treating an elite runner who has an acute hamstring pull. His order includes ice, gentle range of motion exercises, and massage. Which type of massage should you use?
    a. Deep friction
    b. Tapotement
    c. Effleurage
    d. Kneading

13. Indications for the use of high-voltage stimulation in the outpatient physical therapy clinic would include all the following *except:*
    a. Muscle reeducation
    b. Reduction of swelling
    c. Healing of a pressure sore
    d. Increasing circulation in the calf of a patient with thrombophlebitis

14. You are treating a 44-year-old woman who was involved in a car accident, which resulted in a fractured humerus. Due to the severity of the splintered fracture, she sustained nerve damage that involved the forearm musculature. Which type of electrical stimulation would be the best choice to use for her?
    a. Alternating
    b. Direct
    c. Pulsating
    d. It does not matter

15. You notice during an exercise session with a patient who has a brachial plexus injury that you can induce only a very small flicker of a contraction. This response would be rated:
    a. Poor
    b. Poor minus
    c. Trace
    d. Minus trace

16. Which of the following modalities will penetrate 3 to 4 cm of tissue?
    a. Hot pack
    b. Whirlpool
    c. Heating pad
    d. Ultrasound

17. You have observed a patient who has undergone total hip replacement limping in the clinic and you think that she has a weakness of the prime hip abductor. During palpation, which muscle would you observe the most?
    a. Biceps femoris
    b. Sartorius
    c. Gluteus maximus
    d. Gluteus medius
18. Which of the following is a contraindication for cryotherapy?
    a. Burn
    b. Spasm in the rhomboid muscle
    c. Acutely swollen ankle
    d. Raynaud's phenomenon
19. When elbow extension is measured, the axis of the goniometer should be at the:
    a. Medial epicondyle
    b. Lateral epicondyle
    c. Olecranon process
    d. None of the above
20. Fluidotherapy may be administered for all of the following reasons *except:*
    a. To decrease infection
    b. To decrease pain
    c. To increase circulation
    d. To increase range of motion

REFERENCES

1. *Athletic training and sports medicine,* ed 2, Rosemont, Ill., 1990, American Academy of Orthopaedic Surgeons.
2. Hayes K: *Manual for physical agents,* ed 4, Norwalk, Conn., 1993, Appleton & Lange.
3. Prentice WE: *Therapeutic modalities in sports medicine,* St Louis, 1986, Mosby.
4. Gould JA: *Orthopaedic and sports physical therapy,* ed 2, St Louis, 1990, Mosby.
5. Melzack R, Wall PD: Pain mechanisms: a new theory, *Science* 150:971, 1965.
6. Sinaki M: *Basic clinical rehabilitation medicine,* ed 2, St Louis, 1993, Mosby.
7. Daniels L, Worthingham C: *Muscle testing,* ed 3, Philadelphia, 1972, WB Saunders.

SUGGESTED READINGS

Athletic training and sports medicine, ed 2, Rosemont, Ill., 1990, American Academy of Orthopaedic Surgeons.
Daniels L, Worthingham C: *Muscle testing,* ed 3, Philadelphia, 1972, WB Saunders.
Gould JA: *Orthopaedic and sports physical therapy,* ed 2, St Louis, 1990, Mosby.
Hayes K: *Manual for physical agents,* ed 4, Norwalk, Conn., 1993, Appleton & Lange.
Irwin R: *Sports medicine,* Englewood Cliffs, N.J., 1984, Prentice-Hall.
Prentice WE: *Therapeutic modalities in sports medicine,* eds 1 & 2, St Louis, 1986, 1994, Mosby.
Reid D: *Sports injury assessment and rehabilitation,* New York, 1992, Churchill Livingstone.
Sinaki M: *Basic clinical rehabilitation medicine,* ed 2, St Louis, 1993, Mosby.

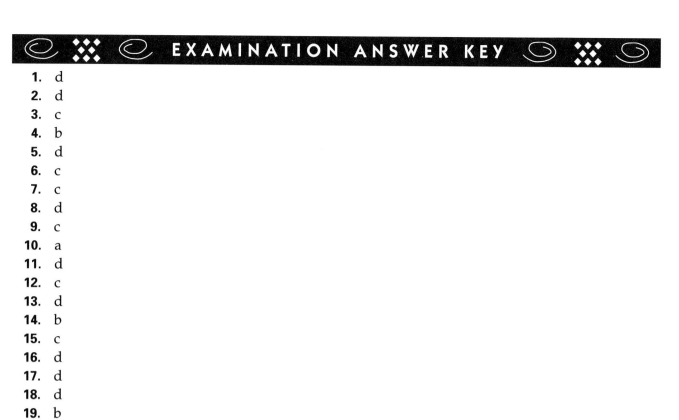

1. d
2. d
3. c
4. b
5. d
6. c
7. c
8. d
9. c
10. a
11. d
12. c
13. d
14. b
15. c
16. d
17. d
18. d
19. b
20. a

EXAMINATION ANSWER SHEET

1. _____

2. _____

3. _____

4. _____

5. _____

6. _____

7. _____

8. _____

9. _____

10. _____

11. _____

12. _____

13. _____

14. _____

15. _____

16. _____

17. _____

18. _____

19. _____

20. _____

EXAMINATION ANSWER SHEET

1. _____

2. _____

3. _____

4. _____

5. _____

6. _____

7. _____

8. _____

9. _____

10. _____

11. _____

12. _____

13. _____

14. _____

15. _____

16. _____

17. _____

18. _____

19. _____

20. _____

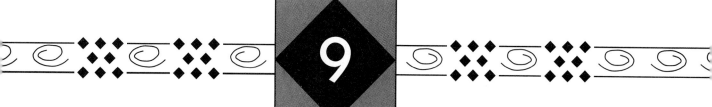

Therapeutic Exercise and Rehabilitation

The goal of every therapeutic exercise regimen is to restore and/or maximize the function of the individual being rehabilitated through a well-planned treatment plan. The treatment planning process involves a series of interrelated steps that lead the physical therapist and assistant to plan and institute a treatment program that will optimally meet the needs of the patient. These steps include:

1. Assessment of the patient's current level of function and degree of dysfunction

2. Establishment of long-term and short-term goals

3. Formulation of an appropriate treatment plan to accomplish these goals

4. Institution of the treatment plan

5. Reassessment of the patient and appropriate adjustment of his/her treatment plan.[1]

This chapter describes some of the most frequently used regimens. For a more comprehensive presentation, the reader is referred to the suggested readings listed at the end of this chapter.

GENERAL CLASSIFICATIONS AND TERMS OF THERAPEUTIC EXERCISE

I. Active exercises are performed by the patient who moves the involved body part independently without any assistance. There are three types of active exercise[2]:

A. Isotonic exercise involves movement through full or partial range of motion in which the muscles contract either concentrically (by shortening) or eccentrically (by lengthening) against resistance (Fig. 9-1).

B. Isometric exercise involves a muscle contraction in which the length of the muscle remains constant while tension develops toward a maximal force against an immovable resistance[3] (Fig. 9-2).

C. Isokinetic exercise involves a muscle contraction in which the speed of motion is at a preset constant velocity. The resistance of the machine accommodates to match the force applied by the body part being tested or rehabilitated. Cybex Corporation manufactures several types of isokinetic equipment (Fig. 9-3).

II. Active-assistive exercises are performed by the patient but require partial assistance by a physical therapist or assistant to complete the exercise. The most common reason for assistance is either weakness in the muscle or joint restriction.

III. Passive exercises are performed when the body part is carried through a full range of motion by a physical therapist or assistant without any help or resistance by the patient.

IV. Self-assistive exercises are performed when a patient has unilateral weakness or involvement and is taught to move the body part through the range of motion using the uninvolved extremity.

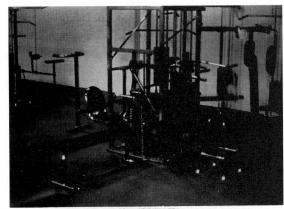

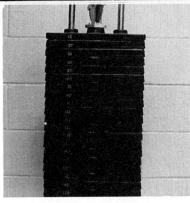

FIG 9-1. Isotonic exercise equipment. (From Prentice WE: *Rehabilitation techniques in sports medicine,* ed 2, St Louis, 1994, Mosby.)

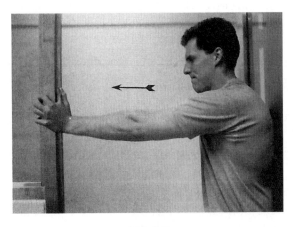

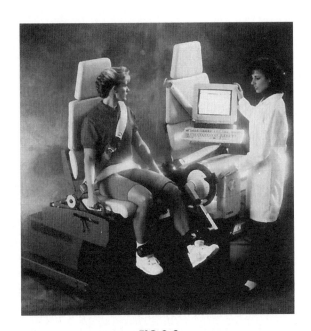

FIG 9-2

FIG 9-3

FIG 9-2. Isometric exercise. (From Prentice WE: *Rehabilitation techniques in sports medicine,* ed 2, St Louis, 1994, Mosby.)

FIG 9-3. Isokinetic exercise equipment. (From Prentice WE: *Rehabilitation techniques in sports medicine,* ed 2, St Louis, 1994, Mosby.)

V. Continuous passive motion (CPM) exercise is exercise that is applied usually by a mechanical device that moves the body part through the range of motion uninterrupted for long periods of time (Fig. 9-4).

VI. Resistive exercises are exercises in which fixed resistance is applied to a muscle as it contracts.
   A. The resistance may be manual or mechanical.
   B. Progressive resistive exercise (PRE) was first described by DeLorme[4] after World War II. He originally recommended a program of progressive resistive exercise that was based on a repetition maximum (RM) of 10. The amount 10 RM is the maximum amount of weight a person can lift 10 times (Table 9-1).

VII. Stretching exercises are performed to increase the stability and mobility of the joints and soft tissue of the body.

◆ **TABLE 9-1**
DeLorme's Program

Set	Amount of Weight	Repetitions
1	50% of 10 RM	10
2	75% of 10 RM	10
3	100% of 10 RM	10

From Prentice WE: *Rehabilitation techniques in sports medicine,* ed 2, St. Louis, 1994, Mosby.

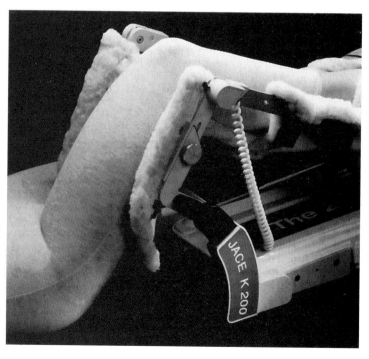

FIG 9-4. Continuous passive motion exercise. (From Prentice WE: *Rehabilitation techniques in sports medicine,* ed 2, St Louis, 1994, Mosby.)

VIII. Closed-kinetic chain exercise involves exercises in which the distal segment of the extremity is fixed (e.g., an exercise performed when the foot is in a weight-bearing position). When the distal segment is stabilized, the kinetic chain is closed[3] (Fig. 9-5). The lower extremity (ankle, knee and hip joints) is more functional in the closed-kinetic chain than in the open-kinetic chain. Although the upper extremity is more functional in the open-kinetic chain, closed-kinetic chain exercise also may be performed for the upper extremity (Fig. 9-6).

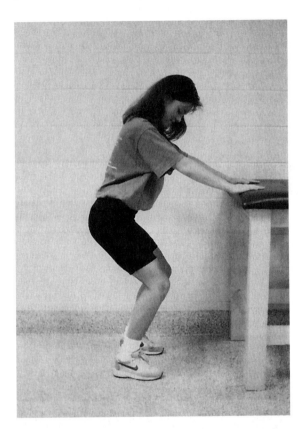

FIG 9-5.   Closed-kinetic chain exercise for lower extremity. (From Prentice WE: *Rehabilitation techniques in sports medicine,* ed 2, St Louis, 1994, Mosby.)

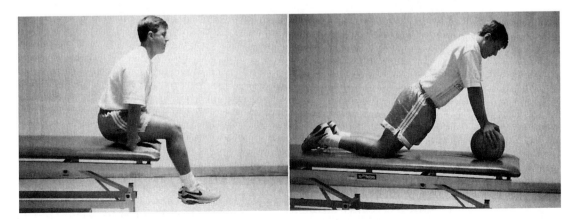

FIG 9-6.   Closed-kinetic chain exercise for upper extremity. (From Prentice WE: *Rehabilitation techniques in sports medicine,* ed 2, St Louis, 1994, Mosby.)

IX. Open-kinetic chain exercise involves exercises in which the distal segment of the extremity is not fixed or weight bearing. Most lower extremity rehabilitation equipment is designed for open-kinetic chain exercise (i.e., knee extension on the Cybex machine; seated knee flexion on Nautilus or Cybex machine).

X. Closed-packed position is the position in which opposing joint surfaces are fully congruent, in maximal contact, and tightly compressed (Table 9-2).

XI. Loose-packed position is the position in which the opposing joint surfaces are not congruent and some parts of the articular capsule are lax. The maximum loose-packed position is the position in which the capsule and its ligaments are the most lax and separation of the joint surfaces is the greatest (Table 9-2).

XII. Specificity of exercise states that exercise training must be relevant to the demands of the sport or the individual's activities of daily living.

XIII. Intensity refers to the degree of work or effort exerted by the patient or athlete.

XIV. Duration is the time it takes to complete the desired exercise.

XV. Frequency is the number of workouts that are performed in a given time (i.e., how many exercise sessions per week).

XVI. Reversibility is basically the "use it or lose it" theory.

XVII. Periodization is a concept that divides an annual training plan into small segments or cycles.

XVIII. Proprioceptive neuromuscular facilitation (PNF) was developed by Herman Kabat, Margaret Knott, RPT, and Dorothy Voss, RPT, to stretch and strengthen selected muscle groups (Figs. 9-7 and 9-8 and Tables 9-3 and 9-4). Three common PNF techniques are:

   A. Contract-relax is a technique used to increase the flexibility of a tight muscle. The body part is moved until resistance is felt, at which point the patient contracts the muscle against resistance, then after the muscle relaxes, it is moved to the next point in the range of motion where resistance is met.

   B. Hold-relax is a technique in which no motion occurs. The patient actively stretches to a comfortable level. Once this stretch level is reached, the patient applies force against the resistance of a partner; therefore an isometric contraction is reached.

   C. Spiral-diagonal pattern is used in the strengthening of weak muscles and improving specific muscle patterns.

◆ **TABLE 9-2**
Joint Positions

Joint	Closed Packed	Loose Packed
Acromioclavicular	Shoulder abducted to 30 degrees	Shoulder in anatomical position
Sternoclavicular	Full shoulder elevation	Shoulder in anatomical position
Glenohumeral	Maximal shoulder abduction and external rotation	55 degrees of shoulder abduction and 30 degrees of horizontal abduction
Elbow		
Radiohumeral	90 degrees of elbow flexion, 5 degrees of supination	Anatomical position
Ulnohumeral	Maximal elbow extension	70 degrees of elbow flexion, 10 degrees of supination
Radiocarpal	Maximal extension and maximal ulnar deviation	Anatomical position
Hip joint	Maximal extension of the hip and maximal external rotation	30 degrees of hip flexion and abduction with slight lateral rotation
Knee joint	Maximal extension and external rotation	25 degrees of knee flexion
Ankle	Maximal dorsiflexion	10 degrees of plantar flexion

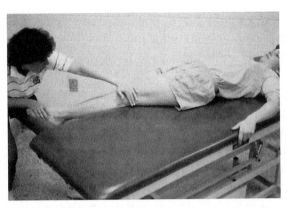

FIG 9-7

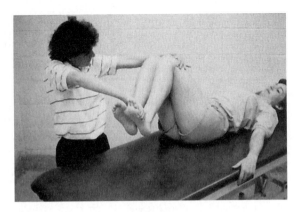

FIG 9-8

FIG 9-7. Lower trunk pattern moving into flexion to the left—starting position. (From Prentice WE: *Rehabilitation techniques in sports medicine,* ed 2, St Louis, 1994, Mosby.)

FIG 9-8. Lower trunk pattern moving into flexion to the left—terminal position. (From Prentice WE: *Rehabilitation techniques in sports medicine,* ed 2, St Louis, 1994, Mosby.)

◆ **TABLE 9-3**
D2 Upper Extremity Movement Patterns

Body Part	Moving into Flexion		Moving into Extension	
	Starting Position	Terminal Position	Starting Position	Terminal Position
Shoulder	Extended	Flexed	Flexed	Extended
	Adducted	Abducted	Abducted	Adducted
	Internally rotated	Externally rotated	Externally rotated	Internally rotated
Scapula	Depressed	Elevated	Elevated	Depressed
	Protracted	Retracted	Retracted	Protracted
	Downwardly rotated	Upwardly rotated	Upwardly rotated	Downwardly rotated
Forearm	Pronated	Supinated	Supinated	Pronated
Wrist	Ulnar flexed	Radially extended	Radially extended	Ulnar flexed
Finger and thumb	Flexed	Extended	Extended	Flexed
	Adducted	Abducted	Abducted	Adducted
Hand position for sports therapist*	Left hand on back of humerus		Left hand on volar surface of humerus	
	Right hand on dorsum of hand		Right hand on cubital fossa of elbow	
Verbal command	Push		Pull	

*For athlete's right arm.
From Prentice WE: *Rehabilitation techniques in sports medicine,* ed 2, St Louis, 1994, Mosby.

XIX. Plyometric exercises use explosive movements to increase strength and power. Commonly performed plyometric exercises include power jumps, leaps and bounds, and throwing a weighted object such as a medicine ball. The main purpose of plyometric exercise is to enhance the excitability of the nervous system for improved reactive ability of the neuromuscular system. Therefore any type of exercise that uses myotatic stretch reflex to produce a more powerful response of the contracting muscle is plyometric in nature.[3]

XX. Buerger-Allen exercises are a series of positional changes in the involved limb that are combined with active foot exercises to increase collateral circulation.

XXI. Frenkel's exercises are a series of exercises developed to treat ataxia for restoration of coordination.

◆TABLE 9-4
D1 Lower Extremity Movement Patterns

Body Part	Moving into Flexion		Moving into Extension	
	Starting Position	Terminal Position	Starting Position	Terminal Position
Hip	Extended	Flexed	Flexed	Extended
	Abducted	Adducted	Adducted	Abducted
	Internally rotated	Externally rotated	Externally rotated	Internally rotated
Knee	Extended	Flexed	Flexed	Extended
Position of tibia	Externally rotated	Internally rotated	Internally rotated	Externally rotated
Ankle and foot	Plantar flexed	Dorsiflexed	Dorsiflexed	Plantar flexed
	Everted	Inverted	Inverted	Everted
Toes	Flexed	Extended	Extended	Flexed
Hand position for sports therapist*	Right hand on dorsimedial surface of foot Left hand on anteromedial thigh near patella		Right hand on lateral plantar surface of foot Left hand on posterolateral thigh near popliteal crease	
Verbal command	Pull		Push	

*For athlete's right leg.
From Prentice WE: *Rehabilitation techniques in sports medicine,* ed 2, St Louis, 1994, Mosby.

PULMONARY REHABILITATION

I. Terminology

Terms	Definitions
1. Apnea	Absence of breathing
2. Bradypnea	Slow rate of breathing
3. Dyspnea	Shortness of breath
4. Tachypnea	Abnormally rapid rate of breathing
5. Tidal volume	Amount of air contained in one breath of inspiration and expiration
6. Residual volume	Amount of air remaining in lungs after full expiration
7. Total lung capacity	Total volume of air in lungs after full inspiration
8. Vital capacity	Maximal amount of air measured on complete expiration after full inspiration

II. Postural drainage positioning[6]
  A. Upper lobes
    1. Apical segments
      a) Patient position: sitting and leaning back against pillow at 30-degree angle (semi-Fowler position)
      b) Action: clap over area between clavicle and top of scapula on each side (Fig. 9-9)
    2. Posterior apical segments
      a) Patient position: sitting and leaning forward over a pillow at a 30-degree angle
      b) Action: stand behind patient and clap over upper back above shoulder blades on both sides (Fig. 9-10)
    3. Anterior segments
      a) Patient position: supine with pillow under knees
      b) Action: clap between clavicle and nipple line on both sides (Fig. 9-11)

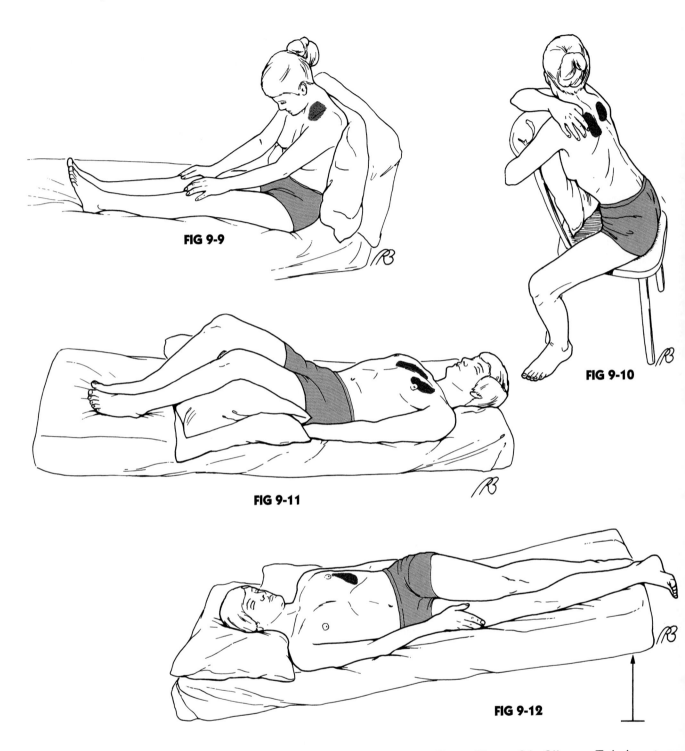

FIG 9-9

FIG 9-10

FIG 9-11

FIG 9-12

FIG 9-9. Postural drainage for apical segments of the upper lobe. (From Shoup CA, Gilmore T: *Laboratory exercises in respiratory care,* ed 3, St Louis, 1988, Mosby.)

FIG 9-10. Postural drainage for the posterior segments of the upper lobes. (From Shoup CA, Gilmore T: *Laboratory exercises in respiratory care,* ed 3, St Louis, 1988, Mosby.)

FIG 9-11. Postural drainage for the anterior segments of the upper lobes. (From Shoup CA, Gilmore T: *Laboratory exercises in respiratory care,* ed 3, St Louis, 1988, Mosby.)

FIG 9-12. Postural drainage for the lingular segment of the left upper lobe. (From Shoup CA, Gilmore T: *Laboratory exercises in respiratory care,* ed 3, St Louis, 1988, Mosby.)

4. Left posterior segment (lingular segment)
   a) Patient position: side lying on right side with head and shoulders on pillows and body turned forward one-quarter turn
   b) Action: clap over left shoulder blade (Fig. 9-12)
5. Right posterior segment
   a) Patient position: side lying on left side rolled forward on a pillow (from shoulders to hips) and body turned one-quarter turn
   b) Action: clap over right shoulder blade (same as Fig. 9-12 but patient lies on left side)
B. Right middle lobe
   1. Patient position: side lying on left side with bottom of bed elevated 14 to 16 inches (Trendelenburg's position)
   2. Action: clap over left nipple (in women, clap under armpit) (Fig. 9-13)
C. Lower lobes
   1. Superior segments: left and right
      a) Patient position: prone with pillow under stomach on flat bed
      b) Action: clap over middle of back on either side of spine (Fig. 9-14)

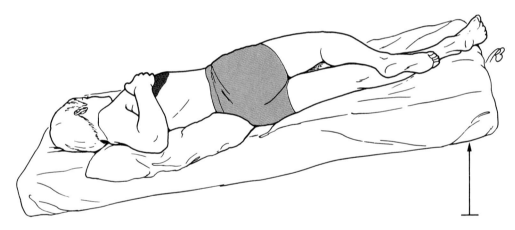

FIG 9-13.   Postural drainage for the right middle lobe. (From Shoup CA, Gilmore T: *Laboratory exercises in respiratory care,* ed 3, St Louis, 1988, Mosby.)

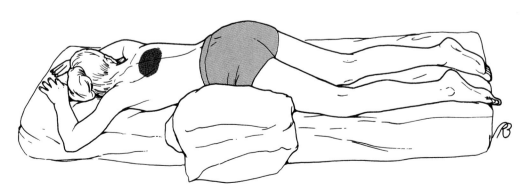

FIG 9-14.   Postural drainage for the superior segments of the lower lobes. (From Shoup CA, Gilmore T: *Laboratory exercises in respiratory care,* ed 3, St Louis, 1988, Mosby.)

2. Lateral basal segment
   a) Patient position: side lying on side opposite one requiring drainage with bottom of bed elevated 18 inches
   b) Action: clap in area of posterior midaxillary line at level of nipple (Fig. 9-15)
3. Anterior basal segment
   a) Patient position: supine with bottom of bed elevated 20 inches
   b) Action: clap at lower ribs on both sides
4. Posterior basal segment
   a) Patient position: prone on stomach with bottom of bed elevated 20 inches
   b) Action: clap at lower ribs on both sides (Fig. 9-16)

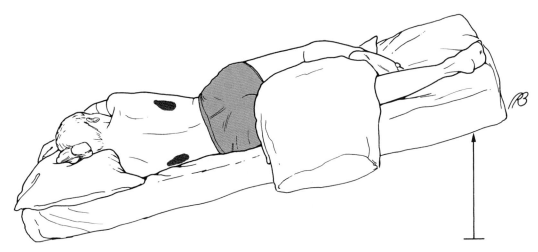

FIG 9-15.   Postural drainage for the lateral basal segment of the lower lobes. (From Shoup CA, Gilmore T: *Laboratory exercises in respiratory care,* ed 3, St Louis, 1988, Mosby.)

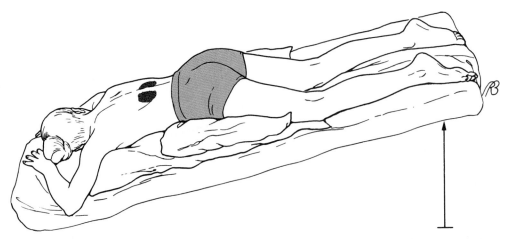

FIG 9-16.   Postural drainage for posterior segments of the lower lobes. (From Shoup CA, Gilmore T: *Laboratory exercises in respiratory care,* ed 3, St Louis, 1988, Mosby.)

CARDIAC REHABILITATION

I. Phases of cardiac rehabilitation
    A. Phase one begins at approximately 3 to 6 days after infarction (or when stable) and lasts until the patient is discharged from the hospital. Activities of this phase include activities of daily living evaluation, vital signs monitoring, and counseling and education of the patient and family. A treadmill test is usually performed before discharge.
    B. Phase two begins with discharge (10 to 14 days) or when patient completes a low-level treadmill test and ends when patient passes the advanced treadmill test. This phase continues the education process and works on building endurance.
    C. Phase three is the long-term follow-up stage. It continues for the rest of the patient's life. The goal is to advance the patient to a point at which he/she can exercise at 75% of the maximum heart rate.

CARDIOPULMONARY RESUSCITATION (CPR)[7]

I. One-rescuer protocol outline for adult victim (establish ABCs)
    A. Airway: head—tilt/chin—lift/jaw—thrust
    B. Breathing: ventilation
    C. Circulation: chest compressions
II. One-rescuer protocol for adult victim
    A. Airway
        1. Shake subject. Responsive? (Fig. 9-17)
        2. Ask subject, "Are you ok?"
        3. Call for help. Contact 911 or Emergency Medical Services when unconsciousness is recognized.
        4. Position subject on back, supporting neck and head. Kneel at subject's shoulders (Fig. 9-18).

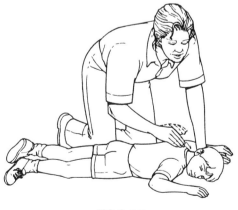

FIG 9-17

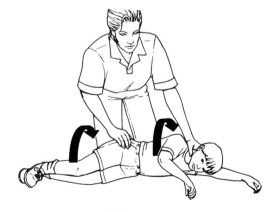

FIG 9-18

FIG 9-17. Tap and shout to check responsiveness. (From American Red Cross: *Community CPR,* St Louis, 1993, Mosby. Courtesy of the American Red Cross. All rights reserved in all countries.)

FIG 9-18. Position victim on back supporting head and neck. (From American Red Cross: *Community CPR,* St Louis, 1993, Mosby. Courtesy of the American Red Cross. All rights reserved in all countries.)

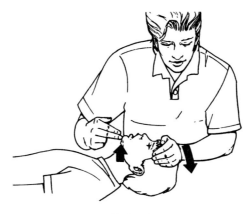

FIG 9-19

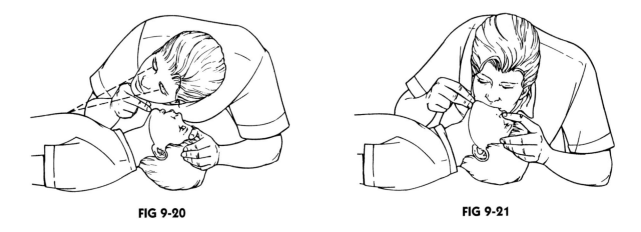

FIG 9-20

FIG 9-21

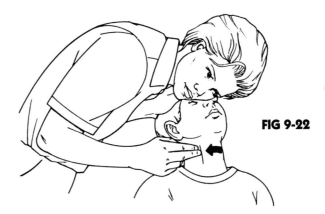

FIG 9-22

FIG 9-19. Tilt the head to open the airway. (From American Red Cross: *Community CPR,* St Louis, 1993, Mosby. Courtesy of the American Red Cross. All rights reserved in all countries.)

FIG 9-20. Listen over the mouth of the victim to check breathing. (From American Red Cross: *Community CPR,* St Louis, 1993, Mosby. Courtesy of the American Red Cross. All rights reserved in all countries.)

FIG 9-21. Pinch the nose and give two slow breaths. (From American Red Cross: *Community CPR,* St Louis, 1993, Mosby. Courtesy of the American Red Cross. All rights reserved in all countries.)

FIG 9-22. Check the pulse. (From American Red Cross: *Community CPR,* St Louis, 1993, Mosby. Courtesy of the American Red Cross. All rights reserved in all countries.)

5. Open airway. Head—tilt/chin—lift (push forehead down and back with palm and lift jaw/chin forward with the other fingers), or jaw—thrust (pull angles of the lower jaw forward and up with each hand on each side while tilting the head back) (Fig. 9-19). (Do not perform head tilt if neck injury is suspected.)

B. Breathing

1. Determine if subject is breathing. Listen over mouth. Does chest rise? Feel air flow (Fig. 9-20).
2. Keep airway open (Fig. 9-20).
3. Pinch nose and perform mouth-to-mouth breathing or other air flow access (Fig. 9-21).
4. Give two breaths, each lasting 1.4 to 2 seconds. Watch chest rise and fall.
5. If breathing is unsuccessful:
   a) Reposition head and ventilate again.
   b) If ventilation is unsuccessful, perform foreign body airway obstruction protocol for the unconscious victim.

C. Circulation

1. Check pulse (usually carotid artery, 5 to 10 seconds) (Fig. 9-22).
2. If there is no pulse, start chest compression.
   a) Place the heel of one hand on the lower one half of the sternum while kneeling at subject's side (Fig. 9-23).
   b) Place the other hand on top of the hand placed on the sternum (Fig. 9-24).
   c) Straighten arms, lock elbows, and place rescuer's shoulders directly over the sternum (Fig. 9-24).
   d) Depress sternum 1½ to 2 inches, and relax, keeping hands on the sternum (Fig. 9-25).

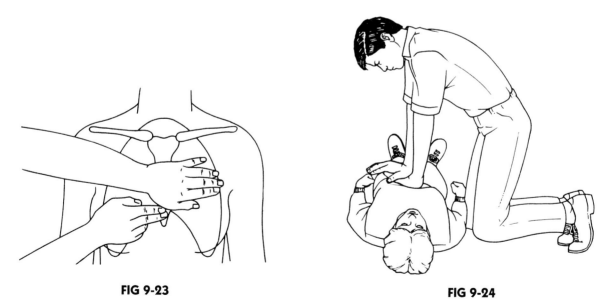

FIG 9-23   **FIG 9-24**

FIG 9-23.   Find the hand position. (From American Red Cross: *Community CPR,* St Louis, 1993, Mosby. Courtesy of the American Red Cross. All rights reserved in all countries.)

FIG 9-24.   Place the other hand on top of the hand on the sternum. (From American Red Cross: *Community CPR,* St Louis, 1993, Mosby. Courtesy of the American Red Cross. All rights reserved in all countries.)

3. Perform 15 compressions over 9 to 11 seconds ("one and two and . . .") at a rate of 60 compressions per minute, including time for respirations (Fig. 9-25).

D. Cycles

    1. Perform four cycles of 15 compressions and two ventilations.
    2. Check pulse (Fig. 9-26).
    3. If there is no pulse, administer two breaths (Fig. 9-27).
    4. Repeat four cycles of 15 compressions and two ventilations.
    5. Check carotid pulse every 2 to 3 minutes.

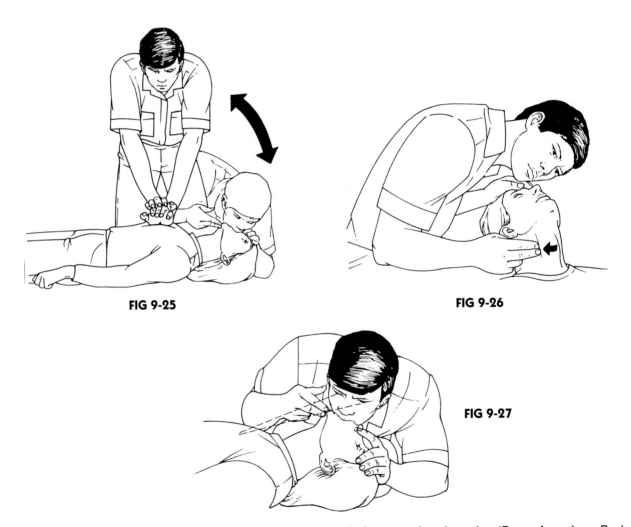

FIG 9-25

FIG 9-26

FIG 9-27

FIG 9-25. Depress the sternum 1½ to 2 inches 15 times and give two slow breaths. (From American Red Cross: *Community CPR,* St Louis, 1993, Mosby. Courtesy of the American Red Cross. All rights reserved in all countries.)

FIG 9-26. Check pulse. (From American Red Cross: *Community CPR,* St Louis, 1993, Mosby. Courtesy of the American Red Cross. All rights reserved in all countries.)

FIG 9-27. Administer two breaths. (From American Red Cross: *Community CPR,* St Louis, 1993, Mosby. Courtesy of the American Red Cross. All rights reserved in all countries.)

III. Two-rescuer protocol for adult victim

ABCs	Compressor	Ventilator
Airway	Position victim	Unresponsive? Open airway
Breathing	Breathing? Does chest rise?	Listen over mouth Give two breaths (1.5 to 2 seconds each)
Circulation	Give five compressions (3 to 4 seconds)	Feel for carotid pulse Give one breath (1.5 to 2 seconds)

Repeat 5:1 cycle 10×
Ventilator checks pulse as needed to assess compressions
Compressor directs switch when needed after ventilation

LOWER EXTREMITY PROSTHETICS

I. Amputation level—terminology

Terms	Definitions
1. Hemicorporectomy	Surgical removal of the pelvis and both lower extremities
2. Hemipelvectomy	Surgical removal of one half (side) of the pelvis and leg
3. Hip disarticulation	Surgical removal of the femur from the pelvis
4. Above-knee amputation	Amputation of the leg above the knee joint
5. Knee disarticulation	Amputation through the joint line of the knee
6. Below-knee amputation	Amputation of the leg below the knee joint
7. Syme's amputation	Amputation of the foot at the ankle joint, including the malleoli
8. Transmetatarsal amputation	Amputation through the midsection of the metatarsals
9. Chopart's amputation	Disarticulation at the midtarsal joint

II. Components and terminology of prostheses
   A. Foot-ankle mechanisms
      1. SACH foot (solid-ankle cushion heel) contains no ankle joint and consists of a cushion heel made of compressed neoprene.
      2. Single-axis foot-ankle contains a carved wooden foot attached to the shank by a single ankle joint. Plantar flexion is limited to 15 degrees and dorsiflexion is limited to 5 degrees. No eversion or inversion is allowed.
   B. Shank systems
      1. Exoskeleton consists of a rigid exterior and outer shell-like construction usually made of laminated plastic.
      2. Endoskeleton refers to an inner, tubular support to which components can be attached. It is used with immediate postoperative prosthetic fits.
   C. Knee components
      1. Single-axis joints allow for flexion-extension. Hyperextension is prevented by the use of an extension stop.
      2. Friction mechanism is provided by an adjustable bushing around the knee bolt. It allows for swing phase control by preventing high heel rise during the first part of swing and terminal swing impact.
      3. Variable friction allows for a more normal gait pattern at faster speeds.
      4. Polycentric knee has more than one axis and therefore allows rotation.
      5. Pneumatic knee is designed to adjust automatically to changes in gait cadence by air escaping through a series of holes.

6. Hydraulic knee is the same as the pneumatic knee but automatic adjustment is allowed by oil escaping through a series of holes.
   D. Socket design
   1. Patellar-tendon bearing socket is named for the major weight-bearing area, the patellar tendon, of the socket.
   2. Quadrilateral socket: above-knee prosthesis is named for the shape of its proximal end. The distal end conforms more to the cone shape of the stump. The quadrilateral shape provides good support and distribution of pressure to the tissues and allows maximum use of the remaining muscles.
   3. Suspension systems function to hold the prosthesis on with close contact between the limb and socket.
III. Gait deviations from prostheses

Deviations	Causes
Lateral trunk bending	Prosthesis too short
	Medial wall of prosthesis too high
	Lateral wall misshaped
Abduction gait (wide walking base)	Prosthesis too long
	Medial wall too high
	Incorrect suspension
	Lateral wall misshaped
	Tight hip abductors
Circumduction	Prosthesis too long
	Knee joint stiff
	Tight hip abductors
	Improper training
	Weak hip flexors
Excessive knee flexion during stance	Prosthesis too long
	Stiff heel cushion
	Foot set in too much dorsiflexion
	Knee flexion contracture
	Weak quadriceps muscle
Rotation of foot on heel strike	Stiff heel cushion
	Malrotation of foot
Vaulting	Prosthesis too long
	Incorrect suspension
	Excessive plantar flexion
	Short residual limb
Forward flexion of trunk	Socket too large
	Hip flexion contracture
	Weak hip extensors

GAIT TRAINING

I. Phases of gait (Fig. 9-28)
   A. Stance phase
   1. *Heel strike:* beginning of stance phase when the heel first contacts the ground (Fig. 9-29)
   2. *Footflat:* immediately following heel strike when the sole of the foot is in contact with the floor (Fig. 9-30)
   3. *Midstance:* point when the body passes directly over the supporting limb (Fig. 9-31)
   4. *Heel-off:* point following midstance when heel leaves the ground (Fig. 9-32)
   5. *Toe-off:* point following heel-off when only the toe of the referenced side is in contact with the ground

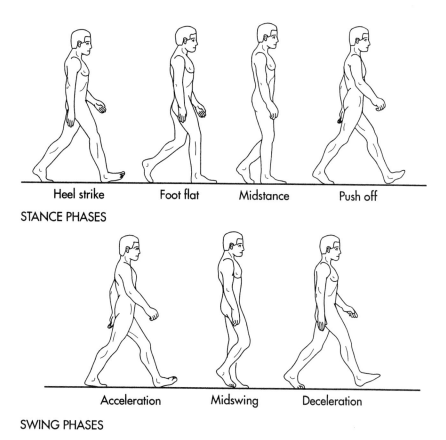

Heel strike   Foot flat   Midstance   Push off

STANCE PHASES

Acceleration   Midswing   Deceleration

SWING PHASES

FIG 9-28. Phases of gait. (From Hartley A: *Practical joint assessment: lower quadrant,* ed 2, St Louis, 1995, Mosby.)

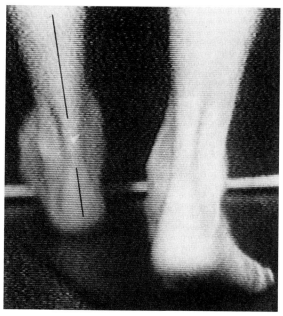

FIG 9-29

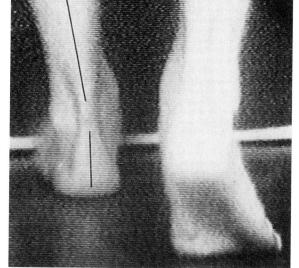

FIG 9-30

FIG 9-29. Left heel strike. (From Gould JA: *Orthopaedic and sports physical therapy,* ed 2, St Louis, 1990, Mosby.)

FIG 9-30. Left footflat. (From Gould JA: *Orthopaedic and sports physical therapy,* ed 2, St Louis, 1990, Mosby.)

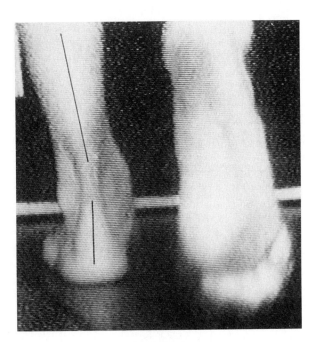

FIG 9-31

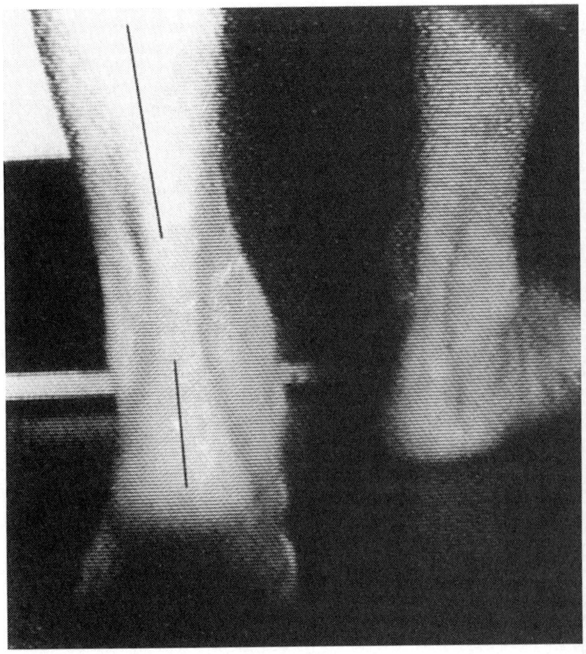

FIG 9-32

FIG 9-31. Normal left midstance. (From Gould JA: *Orthopaedic and sports physical therapy,* ed 2, St Louis, 1990, Mosby.)

FIG 9-32. Left heel-off. (From Gould JA: *Orthopaedic and sports physical therapy,* ed 2, St Louis, 1990, Mosby.)

B. Swing phase (Fig. 9-29)
  1. *Acceleration:* beginning of the swing phase from the time the toe of the referenced leg leaves the ground to the point when the reference leg is directly under the body
  2. *Midswing:* portion of the swing phase when the referenced leg passes directly below the body
  3. *Deceleration:* portion of the swing phase when the referenced leg is decelerating in preparation for heel strike
II. Key muscles involved in gait

Muscle	Action
Quadriceps	Most active during the early stance phase and just before toe-off
Hamstrings	Most active during the late swing phase; key to deceleration
Anterior tibialis	Most active immediately after heel strike to assist in eccentric lowering of the foot (plantar flexion)
Gastrocnemius/soleus	Most active in late stance phase in a concentric raising of the heel during toe-off

REVIEW QUESTIONS

1. During a review of a videotape of the normal gait sequence, which of the components of the stance phase would you *not* expect to find knee flexion?
   a. Heel strike
   b. Footflat
   c. Midstance
   d. Heel-off
   e. Toe-off

2. In one-person mouth-to-mouth artificial respiration, air should be breathed into the individual's mouth at the rate of:
   a. 4 breaths per minute
   b. 8 breaths per minute
   c. 12 breaths per minute
   d. 15 breaths per minute
   e. 20 breaths per minute

3. If you are performing CPR and there is no pulse or respiration, the ratio of heart compressions to breaths is:
   a. 5:1
   b. 1:5
   c. 2:15
   d. 15:2

4. A patient is referred to you complaining of pain in her ankle, which is determined to be due to a tight medial longitudinal arch. Which of the following would be an appropriate stretch?
   a. Anterior tibialis
   b. Extensors of the large toe
   c. Achilles tendon
   d. Posterior tibialis

5. A therapist is helping a patient with a rotator cuff injury to regain the strength in the supraspinatus muscle by the use of the proprioceptive neuromuscular technique of hold-relax. This type of contraction would be:
   a. Isometric
   b. Isotonic
   c. Isokinetic
   d. Concentric

6. Plyometric exercises involve which of the following:
   a. Balance exercises for ataxic patients
   b. Circulatory exercises for the legs
   c. Explosive exercises to increase strength and power
   d. Stretching exercises for cerebral palsy patients

7. Which of the following would be the closed-packed position for the glenohumeral joint?
   a. 180 degrees of shoulder flexion
   b. 30 degrees of shoulder extension
   c. 170 degrees of shoulder abduction and 70 degrees of external rotation
   d. 90 degrees of shoulder flexion

8. Margaret Knott is credited with developing which of the following?
   a. Periodization exercises
   b. Plyometric exercises
   c. Proprioceptive neuromuscular facilitation
   d. Reversibility exercises

9. A physical therapy assistant is treating a pulmonary rehabilitation patient with postural drainage. The area of greatest involvement is the superior segment of the lower right lobe. Which of the following would be the treatment position of choice?
   a. Patient lying on his back with a pillow under his knees
   b. Patient lying on his left side rotated forward 25 degrees
   c. Patient lying on his right side with the foot of the bed elevated 20 inches
   d. Patient lying on his stomach over a pillow

10. Tachypnea is a condition of:
    a. Absence of breathing
    b. Abnormally fast breathing
    c. Abnormally slow breathing
    d. Shortness of breath

11. Which of the following could be used for two-point, three-point, four-point, and swing-through gait?
    a. Straight cane
    b. Quad cane
    c. Walker
    d. Aluminum axillary crutches

12. You are treating an amputee who has an immediate postoperative prosthesis for an above-knee amputation. Which of the following is *not* a benefit of the immediate postoperative prosthesis?
    a. The patient's dressing can be changed daily
    b. It allows for earlier ambulation
    c. It is custom-made for each patient
    d. It helps to form the patient's residual limb

13. A therapist is working with a patient with emphysema and has instructed her to expire maximally after inspiring maximally. In this way the therapist can measure the patient's:
    a. Tidal volume
    b. Residual volume
    c. Total lung capacity
    d. Vital capacity

14. A patient is referred to you for treatment because of decreased circulation in her legs. Which of the following exercises would be the best for the patient?
    a. Frenkel's exercises
    b. Buerger-Allen exercises
    c. Periodization exercises
    d. Plyometric exercises

15. During CPR, how many inches should the sternum be depressed during compressions?
    a. ½ inch
    b. 1 inch
    c. 1½ to 2 inches
    d. 3 inches

16. During CPR, the best location to check the pulse is the:
    a. Brachial artery
    b. Radial artery
    c. Femoral artery
    d. Carotid artery
17. A Syme's amputation is the:
    a. Surgical removal of the pelvis
    b. Surgical removal of the femur
    c. Amputation through the midsection of the midtarsals
    d. Amputation of the foot at the ankle joint, including the malleoli
18. A Chopart's amputation involves:
    a. Amputation of the femur
    b. Amputation of the knee 3 inches below the patella
    c. Amputation at the midtarsal joint
    d. Removal of one half of the pelvis and femur
19. You are seeing a patient who has had surgery on both ankles. She is 50% weight bearing on the right foot and weight bearing as tolerated on the left foot. She also has some problems with balance. Which gait pattern would be the safest for her?
    a. Two-point
    b. Three-point partial weight-bearing
    c. Swing-through
    d. Four-point
20. As a physical therapy assistant, you are instructed to place a patient's hip in the loose-packed position. This position would be:
    a. 30 degrees of hip flexion, 30 degrees of abduction, and 5 degress of external rotation
    b. 90 degrees of hip flexion, 10 degrees of abduction, and 10 degrees of internal rotation
    c. 120 degrees of hip flexion, 30 degrees of abduction, and 30 degrees of internal rotation
    d. 10 degrees of hip extension, 30 degrees of abduction, and 5 degrees of external rotation
21. You are working with a C4 quadriplegic patient. If the medical and nursing staff are not careful to turn patient frequently to relieve pressure on skin, what area is most likely to show skin breakdown?
    a. Iliac crest
    b. Medial condyles
    c. Medial malleolus
    d. Coccyx
22. A patient who has had an MRI study showing a tear of the infraspinatus tendon has been referred to you. Which of the following would you expect to show weakness?
    a. Shoulder external rotation
    b. Shoulder internal rotation
    c. Shoulder adduction
    d. Shoulder abduction
23. A therapist has evaluated a hemiplegic patient with a subluxed shoulder and assigned the patient to you for follow-up care. The therapist placed the patient in a sling, which:
    a. Facilitates the return of normal movement patterns
    b. Prevents recurrence of subluxation
    c. Controls muscle spasticity
    d. Expedites return of muscle strength

24. Which of the following would *not* be a good exercise to teach patient who has undergone total hip replacement surgery 2 weeks ago?
    a. Quadriceps setting
    b. Short arc quads
    c. Hip adductor strengthening
    d. Gentle hip flexion
25. You are giving gait instruction to a below-knee amputee who is having trouble with balance and is laterally bending too much when he walks. The most common cause for this problem is:
    a. Too short a prosthesis
    b. Too long a prosthesis
    c. Tight hip abductors
    d. Too much dorsiflexion in the foot
26. DeLorme devised an exercise program that:
    a. Increases vital capacity
    b. Increases circulation to the lower extremities
    c. Is a progressive resistive exercise program for building strength
    d. Stretches the hamstrings before running
27. The loose-packed position for the ankle is:
    a. 20 degrees of dorsiflexion
    b. 20 degrees of plantar flexion
    c. 10 degrees of dorsiflexion
    d. 10 degrees of plantar flexion

REFERENCES

1. O'Sullivan S: *Physical rehabilitation,* Philadelphia, 1981, FA Davis.
2. Gould JA: *Orthopaedic and sports physical therapy,* ed 2, St Louis, 1990, Mosby.
3. Prentice WE: *Rehabilitation techniques in sports medicine,* ed 2, St Louis, 1994, Mosby.
4. DeLorme T, Wilkins A: Progressive resistance exercise, New York, 1951, Appleton-Century-Crofts.
5. Voight M, Draovitch P: Plyometrics. In Albert, editor: *Eccentric muscle training in sports and orthopaedics,* New York, 1991, Churchill Livingstone.
6. Shoup CA: *Laboratory exercises in respiratory care,* St Louis, 1988, Mosby.
7. *Community CPR,* St Louis, 1993, Mosby.

SUGGESTED READINGS

Athletic training and sports medicine, ed 2, Rosemont, Ill., 1990, American Academy of Orthopaedic Surgeon.
Community CPR, St Louis, 1993, Mosby.
Gould JA: *Orthopaedic and sports physical therapy,* ed 2, St Louis, 1990, Mosby.
O'Sullivan S: *Physical rehabilitation,* Philadelphia, 1981, FA Davis.
Prentice WE: *Therapeutic modalities in sports medicine,* eds 1 and 2, St Louis, 1986, 1994, Mosby.
Shoup CA: *Laboratory exercises in respiratory care,* ed 3, St Louis, 1988, Mosby.
Voight M, Draovitch P: *Plyometrics.* In Albert, editor: *Eccentric muscle training in sports and orthopaedics,* New York, 1991, Churchill Livingstone.

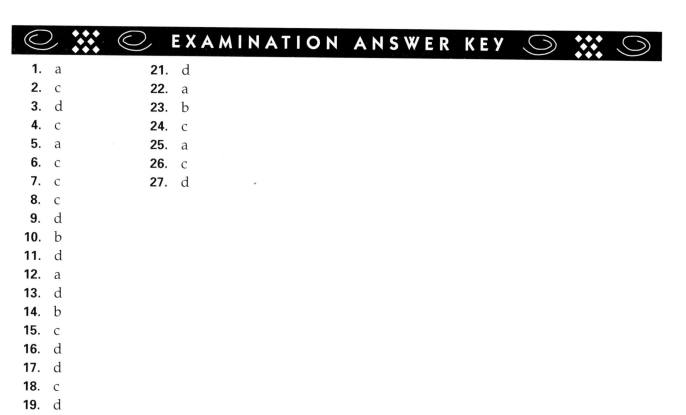

EXAMINATION ANSWER KEY

1.	a	**21.**	d
2.	c	**22.**	a
3.	d	**23.**	b
4.	c	**24.**	c
5.	a	**25.**	a
6.	c	**26.**	c
7.	c	**27.**	d
8.	c		
9.	d		
10.	b		
11.	d		
12.	a		
13.	d		
14.	b		
15.	c		
16.	d		
17.	d		
18.	c		
19.	d		
20.	a		

EXAMINATION ANSWER SHEET

1. _____   21. _____

2. _____   22. _____

3. _____   23. _____

4. _____   24. _____

5. _____   25. _____

6. _____   26. _____

7. _____   27. _____

8. _____

9. _____

10. _____

11. _____

12. _____

13. _____

14. _____

15. _____

16. _____

17. _____

18. _____

19. _____

20. _____

EXAMINATION ANSWER SHEET

1. _____   21. _____

2. _____   22. _____

3. _____   23. _____

4. _____   24. _____

5. _____   25. _____

6. _____   26. _____

7. _____   27. _____

8. _____

9. _____

10. _____

11. _____

12. _____

13. _____

14. _____

15. _____

16. _____

17. _____

18. _____

19. _____

20. _____

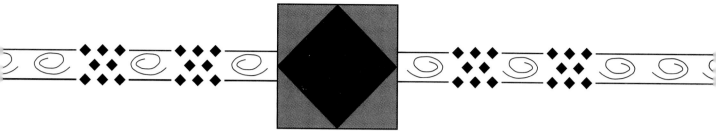

Glossary

a-	prefix meaning *without*
ab-	prefix meaning *deviating from*
abduction	movement away from midline
acid-	prefix meaning *sour*
acr/o-	combining form denoting relationship to an extremity
active insufficiency	inability of a muscle to act (shorten)
acu-	prefix meaning *needle*
ad-	prefix meaning *toward*
adduction	movement toward midline
aden/o-	combining form denoting relationship to gland
adip-	prefix meaning *fat*
afferent fibers	nerve fibers that send impulses from the periphery to the CNS
agonist (prime mover)	muscle that causes motion
alges/i-	combining form denoting oversensitivity to pain
-algia	suffix meaning *pain*
amb/i-	prefix meaning *both sides*
amphiarthrosis joint (cartilaginous)	joint in which two bones are united by either hyaline cartilage or fibrocartilage
an-	prefix meaning *without*
anatomical position	position in which person is standing with feet facing forward, arms at sides, palms facing forward
angi/o-	combining form denoting relationship to vessel
angle of anteversion	angle of the femoral neck in the transverse plane; anterior inclination of the femoral neck
angle of inclination	angle formed by the neck of the femur in the frontal plane
angle of retroversion	reversal of the angle of anteversion in which the femoral neck is angled posteriorly in the transverse plane
angular motion	motion around an axis of rotation in which parts move through same angle and in same direction at the same time but not for same distance
ankyl/o-	combining form meaning *stiff*
antagonist	muscle whose action is opposite of that of agonist
ante-	prefix meaning *before*
anterior	toward front
appendicular skeleton	bones of limbs and their girdles

arachnoid	very thin second layer of the meninges
arthr/o-	combining form denoting relationship to a joint
articular cartilage	thin layer of hyaline cartilage covering bone where it forms a bone
audi/o-	combining form denoting relationship to hearing
aut/o-	prefix meaning *self*
avulsion fracture	fracture in which a piece of bone is pulled loose at the attachment of a tendon
axial skeleton	bones of the skull, hyoid, vertebral column and rib cage
axis of rotation	imaginary line around which a body part rotates
axon	single branch from cell body that takes nerve impulses away from the cell body
bi-	prefix meaning *two, double*
bi/o-	combining form denoting relationship to life
biomechanics	mechanical principles related to body
bipennate muscle	muscle with fasciculi on both sides of central tendon
blast/o-	combining form denoting relationship to cell
brachi/o-	combining form meaning *upper arm*
brady-	combining form meaning *slow*
brainstem	portion of the brain consisting of the midbrain, pons, and medulla oblongata
bronch/o-	combining form denoting relationship to bronchi
burs/o-	combining form denoting relationship to bursa
calcane/o-	combining form denoting relationship to the heel
cancellous (spongy) bone	porous, spongy inside part of bone
capitulum	eminence on the distal end of the lateral epicondyle of the humerus
carcin/o-	combining form meaning *cancer*
cardi/o-	combining form denoting relationship to the heart
carpal tunnel syndrome	pressure and constriction of the median nerve at the wrist
caudal	closer to the tail or feet
-cele	suffix meaning *herniation*
center of mass	point at which all the body's mass is concentrated or the balance point for the body
central sulcus	groove that separates the frontal and parietal lobes
cephalic	closer to the head
cerebellum	posterior portion of the brain attached to the brainstem at the pons; it functions to maintain muscle tone, balance and coordination of movement
cerebr-	combining form denoting relationship to the cerebrum
cerebrum	largest and main portion of the brain; it is responsible for the highest mental functions
chir/o-	combining form denoting relationship to the hand
chondr/o-	combining form denoting relationship to the cartilage
circumduction	combination of flexion, extension, abduction, and adduction
closed-packed position	joint position in which there is maximum contact between the two joint surfaces and the ligaments are taut
compact bone	hard, dense outer shell of bone
concentric contraction	muscle contraction in which the muscle contracts and the muscle attachments move toward each other

condyl/o-	combining form denoting relationship to a rounded process
contractility	ability to shorten or contract (produce tension)
corpus callosum	largest commissure (connection) of the brain connecting the cerebral hemispheres
cost/o-	combining form denoting relationship to the ribs
cox-	combining form denoting relationship to the hip joint
coxa valga	deformity of the hip in which there is an increase in the angle of inclination of the femoral neck (greater than 125 degrees)
coxa vara	deformity of the hip in which there is a decrease in the angle of inclination of the femoral neck (less than 125 degrees)
cry/o-	combining form denoting relationship to cold
curvilinear motion	linear motion in a straight line but in a curved path
deep	away from the surface
dendrite	branching extension of cell body that receives information and transmits the information to the cell body
derm/o-	combining form denoting relationship to the skin
diaphysis	shaft of the bone
diarthrosis (synovial) joint	joint with no direct union between the two bones; joint cavity is filled with fluid
dis-	prefix meaning *apart, separation*
distal	away from the trunk
dorsal	toward the back (posterior)
dorsiflexion	ankle movement of the foot toward the shin or wrist movement of the dorsum of the hand posteriorly
dura mater	most superficial and thickest layer of the meninges
dynam-	combining form meaning *power* or *strength*
dynamic	moving
-dynia	combining form meaning *pain*
dys-	combining form meaning *difficult*
eccentric contraction	lengthening contraction in which muscle attachments separate
ect/o-	prefix meaning *outer*
-ectomy	suffix meaning *removal*
edema	swelling
efferent fibers	nerve fibers that send impulses from the CNS to the periphery
elasticity	ability to recoil or return to resting length
endomysium	sheath surrounding each muscle fiber
endosteum	tissue lining inner cavities of bone
epiphysis	end of the bone
equilibrium	balanced state in which there is no movement because the sum of all the forces and torques acting on the object is zero
erythr/o-	combining form meaning *red*
extensibility	ability to stretch or lengthen when force is applied
extension	straightening movement (increase the joint angle)
external rotation (lateral)	movement of the anterior surface toward the midline
eversion	turning the sole of the foot outward at the ankle

facet	small, flattened articular surface
faci-	combining form meaning *face*
fibr/o-	combining form denoting relationship to fibers
flat bone	thin, curved bone consisting of two layers of cancellous bone
flexion	bending movement (or decrease the joint angle)
fossa	depression
fundamental position	position in which a person is standing with feet facing forward, arms at sides, and palms facing the sides of the body
fusiform muscle	spindle-shaped muscle that is wider in the middle and has tendons on both ends
gangli/o-	combining form denoting relationship to a nerve cell
genu valgum	condition of the knees in which the knees are abnormally close (knock knees)
genu varum	a condition of the knees in which the knees are abnormally far apart (bowlegs)
gon/io-	combining form denoting relationship to an angle
hemi-	prefix meaning *half*
hem/o-	combining form denoting relationship to the blood
horizontal abduction	movement in which the shoulder is flexed to 90 degrees and then abducted
horizontal adduction	movement in which the shoulder is flexed to 90 degrees and then adducted
hydr/o-	combining form denoting relationship to water
hypo-	prefix meaning *under, less than*
hypothenar eminence	ridge on the palm on the ulnar side created by the intrinsic muscles of the little finger
inferior	below or lower than another structure
infra-	prefix meaning *below, under*
internal rotation (medial)	movement of the anterior surface toward the midline
inversion	turning the sole of the foot inward at the ankle
irritability	ability to respond to a stimulus
isokinetic contraction	muscle contraction in which the muscle shortens at a constant speed and tension is maximal over the full range of motion
isometric contraction	muscle contraction in which the muscle produces a constant tension and the muscle length remains the same
isotonic contraction	muscle contraction in which the muscle produces a constant tension and the muscle shortens in length
-itis	suffix meaning *inflammation*
kinematics	time, space, and mass aspect of motion
kinesiology	scientific study of human movement
kinetics	forces that cause movement
labrum	ring of fibrocartilage around shoulder and hip joints that increases the depth of the joint cavity
lateral	away from the midline
lateral fissure	deep fold that separates the temporal lobe from the rest of the cerebrum
lateral flexion	movement of the trunk sideways

linea (line)	low ridge
linear (translatory) motion	motion that occurs in a straight line; movement occurs in different regions of same body part at the same distance, same direction, and same time
long bone	tubular-shaped bone in which its length is greater than its width
loose-packed position	joint position in which there is less than maximum contact between the two joint surfaces and the contact areas are frequently changing
lys/o-	combining form meaning *destruction of*
macr/o-	combining form meaning *large, enlarge*
malac/o-	combining form meaning *softening*
medial	toward the midline
medulla oblongata	most inferior portion of the brainstem; it is the center for reflexes of regulation of heart rate, coughing, breathing, swallowing, sneezing, vomiting, and blood vessel diameter
medullary cavity	large cavity within the diaphysis
multipennate muscle	muscle with many tendons and fibers in between
myositis ossificans	condition in which bone deposits are laid down in soft tissue, which causes ossification in the muscle
neutralizer	muscle that prevents unwanted motion
node of Ranvier	short interval or break in the myelin sheath of a nerve fiber between Schwann cells
osteoblast	cell that produces the bone matrix
osteocyte	bone cell surrounded by bone matrix
palmar flexion	flexion of the wrist
passive insufficiency	inability of a muscle to lengthen any farther without injury
periosteum	connective tissue membrane covering the outer surface of bone except where articular cartilage is present
pes cavus	high-arched foot
pes planus	flat foot
pia mater	third meningeal layer, which is bound tightly to the surface of the brain and spinal cord
plane of motion	two-dimensional flat surface running through an object; motions occur either in the plane or parallel to the plane
plantar flexion	movement of the foot toward the plantar surface
posterior	toward the back
pronation	rotation of the palm so that it faces posteriorly
protraction	movement anterior or away from the midline
proximal	closer to the trunk
radial deviation	movement of the hand laterally from the anatomical position toward the radial side of the wrist
rectilinear motion	linear motion in a straight line
red marrow	site of blood cell production
retraction	movement posterior or toward the midline
rhomboid muscle	flat, four-sided muscle with broad attachments

sesamoid bone	oval-shaped bone found within tendons
spondylolisthesis	forward displacement of one vertebra over another caused by a bilateral defect of the pars interarticularis
spondylolysis	fatigue fracture or defect of the posterior neural arch of the vertebrae at the pars interarticularis
stabilizer	muscle that supports and allows the agonist to work
static	nonmoving
superficial	toward the surface
superior	above or higher than another structure
supination	rotation of the palm so that it faces anteriorly
synapse	gap between nerve cells that transmits impulses from one cell to another cell
synarthrosis (fibrous) joint	Joint in which two bones are united by fibrous tissue
synergist	muscle that works together with another muscle to cause movement
tenodesis	tendon action of a muscle (stretch)
thalamus	major sensory relay center; it influences mood and movement and is the pain perception center
torque	rotation that results from a force that is not applied through the center of mass
triceps surae muscle	combination of the gastrocnemius and soleus muscles
ulnar deviation	movement of the hand medially from the anatomical position toward the ulnar side of the wrist
valgus force	lateral force
varus force	medial force
ventral	toward the belly (anterior)
winged scapula	outward tilting of the vertebral border of the scapula caused by weakness of the serratus anterior muscle
yellow marrow	fat stored within the medullary cavity

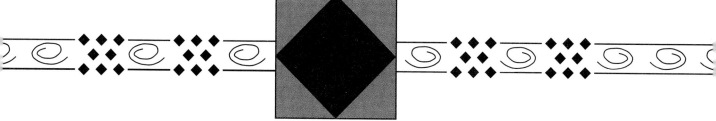

Index